TWO ANGEL WINGS

A Mother Daughter Story of Love and Inspiration

Arlene Webster

ISBN 0-7414-3780-5

Published by:

INFINITY
PUBLISHING.COM

1094 New DeHaven Street, Suite 100
West Conshohocken, PA 19428-2713
Info@buybooksontheweb.com
www.buybooksontheweb.com
Toll-free (877) BUY BOOK
Local Phone (610) 941-9999
Fax (610) 941-9959

Printed in the United States of America

Printed on Recycled Paper

Published January 2007

In Memory of

Stephanie Rae Stanich

CONTENTS

INTRODUCTION

Although my daughter Nancy's Harrington Rod spinal surgery for scoliosis took place many years ago, the decisions we had to make and the emotions and fears we experienced then are the same as parents and their children face today.

Scoliosis remains a very serious issue and more prevalent than many realize, especially for young teenage girls.

There still is no known prevention.

There still is no known cure.

There have been many inroads made in surgery - different procedures, different types of rods, and most importantly, the fact that patients no longer spend months in casts and many more in braces. Even so, it remains just as serious, just a scary, just as emotional.

It would have been easy to censure ourselves or lament to God, "Why this? Why our child?" We tried so hard not to. God usually has his reasons and hands them out it due time. My faith assures me that this is the way He works.

With our faith in God's love and the surgeon's skill, we endured Nancy's extensive surgery, her months in casts, days when there were hints of depression, exhaustion and her impatience to get on with life.

Nancy's life continues to be a full and happy one, with a loving and supportive husband, talented and beautiful daughter, wonderful son-in-law and two precious grandsons.

I don't even want to think about how it would have been had she not made the decision to say "yes."

My hope is that all parents and their children faced with the diagnosis of scoliosis and the necessity to make the decision to have surgery will find the faith and courage to do their research, trust their doctors and themselves, and make the right decision.

PROLOGUE

Two Angel Wing shells rest in a black shell box on the divider in my living room. Two Angel Wings, taking center spot amidst other shells my daughter, Nancy, and I collected from our vacation island in the Gulf of Mexico the summer she turned eighteen.

Perfect?

No. In fact, they aren't even a pair. Both are left Angel Wings, the ribs all going in the same direction. No matter. We shall always treasure them.

When I was little, I believed I had a Guardian Angel, as each child is said to have. I was sure she hovered over me, protecting and loving, touching my forehead when it was feverish and keeping watch while I slept.

As we grow older, much of our spontaneous faith may be lost. A now sophisticated world has conditioned us to hide any child-like ways for fear we may be considered immature. We think we must not shatter the illusion of self-sufficiency we have developed. Fight it though we try, a bit of the child does remain and the need, once in a while, to feel protected.

It is my belief that because we are less than perfect in an imperfect human world, we can never grow so sure, so self-reliant that we do not at times lean toward someone or something. I believe God is our supreme strength. Yet, as the Bible shows us, it is the Angel who is His messenger, ministering directly. With her two Angel wings she can fly from Him to us in time to save, guide, or comfort in any hour.

A childish fantasy? Perhaps.

Our two Angel Wing shells are proof of that faith, a faith I hope Nancy and I never lose.

TWO ANGEL WINGS

CHAPTER ONE

Surgery

There are certain days in our lives that stand out beyond all others. For my husband, Fred, and me, July ninth, 1965 was one.

The day began early. Before sunrise I shut off the alarm, although there had been no need to set it. I'd been awake for hours, lying in the quiet, thinking. Fred still slept and I decided not to disturb him just yet. The day would be long enough.

I arose, put on my robe and slippers and tiptoed into the hall. Our daughter Nancy's door was open. Open before daybreak after so many years of being closed. Each morning I would knock and say, "Time to get up. You'll be late for school!" Or, "Wake up, Nan. Stephanie will be here before you've even had breakfast!"

Not today. Today there would be no usual routine, no usual anything. Nancy was done with her schooling for awhile and she wouldn't be going anywhere with Steph for many months to come. I stood in her doorway and glanced beyond to the emptiness. The hall light played on the big double bed made up neatly with its white hobnailed bedspread. The whole room was neat and empty and all too quiet.

Turning from the emptiness, I went straight down the hall to the kitchen, trying to push worry aside on the way. Worry only led to exhaustion. From here on in I knew I would need all my strength.

Soon my iron skillet was sputtering and sizzling with frying bacon. I had little appetite, but knew I needed to eat something. I hoped Fred would eat too. We had a long day ahead of us. Nancy was scheduled for eight a.m. Harrington Rod surgery to correct the 50-degree thoracic / 70-degree lumbar curves in her spine. We planned to be at the hospital long before that.

From my kitchen window I could see not one light on anywhere on our street. I squeezed oranges, made toast, set the table, then stood before the window again. There were several lights on now. Our world was slowly waking up.

The ficus tree on our front lawn was barely visible as the hint of morning began in the eastern sky. In the eight years we had lived here the tree had grown like Nancy. One day a tiny sproutling, then whoosh, up, up, reaching for the sky as we reached for our dreams. But now, our dreams would have to wait.

"Hey." Fred's voice snapped me back to the kitchen. "Don't burn my bacon." He entered the room and gave me one of his bear hugs. I felt the comfort of his presence, his quiet strength.

The sun was just above the horizon as we started the twenty-five miles to Miami's Variety Children's Hospital. We rode in silence. There were times when words were unnecessary. I sat close to Fred, feeling the warmth of his shoulder, feeling the love we both had for our child transmitted from him to me as if in one being.

When we arrived at the hospital, Nancy's door was closed and we were asked to remain outside for a few minutes until the prepping for surgery was completed. Fred leaned against the wall opposite her door. I stood beside him. One minute. Two. Five. We waited.

"It's all right to go in now." A figure in starched white hurried out and past us.

We entered and saw our seventeen-year-old daughter leaning back on white hospital sheets. She saw us and propped herself up on one elbow.

"Hi, mom. Hi, dad."

"How goes it?" Fred asked.

"Fine, dad."

I kissed Nancy's forehead and sat on the side of her bed. Fred pushed a chair close and sat down. We each held one of her hands, something she would never have allowed under ordinary circumstances. At nearly eighteen you simply didn't hold hands with your parents. Today she didn't mind though.

She squeezed our hands, then looked up at the ceiling as she leaned back against the pillow. "Ooee. I feel as if I'm floating."

The relaxant was taking effect. Words said now would drift away. She wouldn't remember. Nevertheless we talked. Nancy most of all, chattering on as if she were the most vibrant of conversationalists.

"Stephanie was here after you guys left last night. You know how Steph is. She had me laughing 'til my stomach got sore. The nurses spoke to her, but I told her not to mind them."

We nodded. She continued, her voice softer and her run on words a bit slurred.

"Oh, mom, dad. Dr. Keiser is so nice. He really is. The nurses are a little scared of him 'cause he won't stand for any mistakes. But all the kids love him."

We heard a squeaking sound and looked toward the door. The moment we dreaded had arrived. Two aides rolled a narrow stretcher in and alongside the bed. One of the nurses entered and tucked Nancy's hair up into a surgical cap until every wisp was out of sight.

"There now," she said, squeezing Nancy's arm. "You're ready for a grand entrance."

Fred and I let go of Nancy's hands and stepped back out of the way.

The aides echoed the nurse's theme, "Come on, honey," they said. "Let's get this show on the road."

With quick, efficient hands they transferred Nancy from the bed to the stretcher. We followed, as they wheeled Nancy out into the hall, then walked alongside as far as we were allowed.

Fred leaned over first and took her hand. "Your mom and I will be right here. See you in a little while. Okay?" He kissed the top of her head.

"Okay, dad," Nancy's words came out slowly.

Fred stepped back and I went to her, praying I wouldn't cry. What could I say? I touched her cheek. Flushed and warm, her face was a contrast to the whiteness of her hospital gown and sheets. White. White like the two Angel Wing shells in the shell box in our living room.

I leaned over and whispered, "Remember."

"What, mom?" she asked, groggy from the medication.

"The two Angel Wings," I said.

She smiled, looked up at her dad and me and whispered, "Two Angel Wings."

The aides nodded, then continued to push the stretcher through the double doors leading to the surgery wing where Dr. Keiser was waiting.

When the doors swung shut behind Nancy, Fred and I stood there without moving. Although we were together, a feeling of aloneness overwhelmed me. I wanted to reach out to him, but instead remained frozen in one spot. As I looked down the hall where our daughter had been wheeled, a terror I had never experienced before threatened to envelop me. A strange feeling of being not one, but two people. The real me standing in the middle of a hospital corridor, the other viewing the whole incident from a distance, as if it were all a bad dream.

I closed my eyes for a few moments, trying to bring the two parts of me together and into control. Fred touched my arm and spoke softly, "Come on, let's sit down."

He led me to a chair in one of the waiting rooms of Taylor Pavilion, then sat down beside me. His quiet, calm manner was comforting. At that moment I didn't want to talk or even think.

I fingered magazines, then stared down at the terrazzo floor. Nearby, elevator doors opened and closed with people going down, others coming up. Nurses and doctors passed by. Parents arrived and sat near us. They spoke to each other in hushed tones, then smiled at us. We smiled back. Understanding smiles with an instant bond. We were bound by love for a child. They for theirs. We for ours.

Time passed slowly. The clock ticked forward to nine. Over an hour since we had seen our daughter disappear beyond the swinging doors.

I couldn't forget Dr. Keiser's words, "There is no going back once the surgery is performed."

What was happening to Nancy at this moment? How far had the surgery proceeded? Although he had outlined the surgery in detail, I could only marvel at the skill in his hands. Skill that could insert steel rods to straighten a child's spine, then fuse the vertebrae to hold the spine straight. It was almost too much to comprehend.

I looked down at my own hands. They could cook, sew, garden. Once they played a violin quite well. They always had a love for writing, but...

Fred leaned over nudging my arm, "How about a cup of coffee?"

In the hospital cafeteria, we welcomed the sound of rattling dishes and banging trays. People going through every day motions. We stood in line, filled our cups, then sat down at one of the tables. I had little desire to talk, but let the sounds of the room surround me. Bits of conversation. Laughter. To be amidst normal activity felt good. It reassured me. We sat, sipping our coffee until our cups were empty, than stood to go back upstairs.

The next hour we spent walking the halls of the hospital. We tried sitting in one waiting room, then another. We picked up and looked at magazine after magazine, putting each one down without remembering what we read. I found myself in bewilderment, wondering the hows and whys. What could possibly have caused such severe curves in Nancy's spine? Had I done something wrong? I had to know why. Somehow I knew I must find answers. If there were any.

Two hours had passed when one of Dr. Keiser's assisting doctors approached us.

"Mr. and Mrs. Webster?"

"Yes?" Fred replied and we stood up.

"Dr. Keiser asked me to tell you that your daughter, Nancy, is doing well so far."

"Thank you," we both echoed.

Looking straight at me the doctor said, "May I say you look very concerned, Mrs. Webster."

"Yes, doctor, I am," I admitted.

"Please. Be assured we are right here, ready to keep you informed on everything you need to know."

"Thank you," Fred said.

The doctor continued, "By the way, lunch is served from eleven to two. Why don't you both go down when you feel like it, get something to eat and join the other families? If there is any more news we will find you." He turned and hurried back to surgery.

With still another hour before the cafeteria opened for lunch we wondered, each to ourselves, how to fill the time. My six foot three Fred wanted to take a walk, needing to stretch his long legs.

"Do you mind?" he asked.

"No. Of course not," I answered.

My thoughts were only of Nancy. Her smile. The way she lowered her blue eyes when she spoke. Her assurance on a horse. The way her hair few back when she urged her horse into a canter, making him follow her every signal, horse and rider in complete harmony. Attuned the way we all should be in life. Responding, rather than backing off. Loving and understanding, rather than hurting one another.

Life was like riding a horse. You could control the horse, or the horse could control you. The choice was yours. Only by pushing yourself forward with firmness of decision could you direct its path. Nancy had made a difficult decision that would direct her path for the rest of her life.

My mind went back to the two Angel Wing shells in the shell box at home. Two Angel Wings to fly with faith and lift men's souls. To lift my soul. At the mere thought of them, warmth filled me. I knew God was watching over Nancy. He was guiding the surgeon's hands. The two Angel Wings were my proof.

Memories of our recent week on Sanibel Island filled my head. Nancy had made that one of the conditions for going through with surgery. As my mind drifted, it seemed as if I was being transported back to our island. I could feel the warmth of the sun on my back; the sand sifting between my toes.

CHAPTER TWO

A Time to Forget

The first thing we couldn't help mentioning was the sea. It hit the beach with a force we hadn't seen in years and left foamy swirls as it receded. We stood at the edge, sandals in hand, trying to take in everything at once; the gray churning waters of the Gulf, the cloud filled sky, the shell strewn beach.

There is a timelessness about the sea that makes the adult feel childlike. The past, present and future seem to melt into one moment. There is a feeling of infinity in its constant motion. Although we weren't native to the island, several summers of vacationing here made us feel a part of it.

We were home!

Smash! Another breaker covered our legs, frothed at our knees and spit at our shorts. Laughing, we stepped backward and turned away from the fury.

"Wow! Neat!" Nancy exclaimed. "They're really coming in! We should find some great shells this year!"

I smiled as I watched her beaming young face, her eyes alive with delight.

After a four-hour drive from Miami, the salt spray felt good on my hot cheeks. We squiggled our toes into the wet sand and soon, back and forth like two children, we played with the sea.

On one turn toward shore I stopped, realizing the heaps of shells usually ridging the high water mark were now only a small scattering in a line above me. Strange, I thought.

Years before an islander had said to me, "Wait and see. If they build the causeway and bridge, it will ruin everything."

"I hope not," I had responded. "There is too much of what life is all about right here."

Each summer Nancy and I did try to go back, hoping nothing had changed. We would wait in line to board the old ferry for the ride across the bay. The pelicans were always there to greet us. We enjoyed the seclusion of our beach-combing days and quiet nights. Time for mother and daughter to connect. On Sanibel we became kin to the sand, the sea and the slower pace of life. During our week we would walk the beach, hunting for shells during the day. At night we would sit on our balcony, listening to the sounds of the sea, later letting its calming rhythm lull us to sleep.

We wanted this year to be the same. I knew in my heart it couldn't be. Like the island's turning point, there was also one in our lives. No amount of trying could change any of it.

On the island things had already begun to change. A causeway and bridge now stretched from the mainland to the island's shore. Minutes before, Nancy had driven my car past Punta Rassa Road leading to the old ferry dock. Instead of turning down the road as we used to, we stopped to pay our toll, then continued onto the new causeway and bridge cutting its way through the once free waters.

It was hard not to look back and remember. The old ferry dock was barely visible beyond the overgrowth. A few pelicans still sat atop the pilings, but the dock was empty. The ferry was gone. There would be no waiting in line for our turn to drive onto the ferry. No toot of the horn as it cleared the pilings and picked up speed. There would be no standing on the bow letting spray whip our cheeks as the ferry plowed through three miles of open water and we left the real world behind.

My game with the sea finished, I turned back to face it. Under the late afternoon sky the waters were changing colors. Off in the distance came the sound of faint rumbles. On the horizon, thunderheads were building up and moving toward land, darkening the water to gray-green.

"Come on, Nan. We'd better get unpacked." I pointed skyward.

"Plenty of time, mom!" Nancy's reply held the casualness of her seventeen years. She wiggled her toes in the foam. Toes I had watched grow to take their first steps. Toes to stand tiptoe on to reach the dolls on her closet shelf. Toes to fit into the stirrups of a horse's saddle. Five days ago those toes had pointed her way across the platform where she received her high school diploma.

This year we came to the island with more than the usual snorkel, fins and diving mask for Nancy, books, typewriter and sunglasses for me. We came with a void to be filled by the sea and its constancy, its reassurance of the continuity of life and hope. We came knowing that after Nancy's impending spinal surgery, she would be homebound for almost a year.

On the drive over, her only comment about it had been, "Let's not talk about it this week."

"It's a deal."

"Promise?"

"Promise," I repeated. But I knew neither of us would stop thinking about it.

Another rumble reached us. A sudden gust of wind whipped at my blouse.

"Come on, Nan. We've got a lot of stuff to get up to the apartment. How would my new sun hat look all soggy wet?"

"Oh, mom! It's not going to rain yet!" She turned from me and rushed toward another breaker.

Oh, well. This week was a special one. The memories we made here would have to last us a long time. I left Nancy at the water's edge and headed up toward the beach path alone, my toes digging into the wet sand and then into fluffy dryness. When I reached the high tide line I turned and stood waiting for her.

Waiting. There would be so much of that ahead of us. I'd better get used to it. Nancy would also, but not just yet. Give her time. Her own time.

A close crash of thunder sent her skipping out of the water toward me.

"Ready?" I asked.

"Ready, mom." She swung her sandals back and forth on two fingers, her face aglow.

Youth. So beautiful. So fresh and tender. Yet, at the same time, so determined.

Nancy was right. We did make it to the second floor studio apartment with all our stuff in plenty of time. Supper was easy. Hamburgers and salad on paper plates with cups of cold milk. We took our meal out to the balcony where we could watch the storm approach.

Nancy sat with her slim legs outstretched, her bare feet resting on the railing. As she balanced her plate on her lap, I visualized her salad whooshing off onto the redwood floor. I set my plate on the table beside me, not as sure as Nancy of my ability to balance it on my lap.

"Wow! Did you see that?" Nancy pointed her fork skyward. A bolt of lightening ripped down out of the dark clouds off shore, piercing the deep gray waters. Thunder was still rolling when another bolt zigzagged down. A sheet of rain obscured the horizon and resembled a massive curtain on a gray stage. Instead of moving aside, it began moving forward. We watched in awe as it came toward us, first blocking out the ocean, then the shoreline, then finally the beach path.

Wind whipped through the palms near the balcony. Another crash. We decided it was time to go in and close the French doors against the beating rain and wind. As we finished dinner we talked about the week ahead. The shelling we would do, swimming, walking the beach and the books and writing I hoped to catch up on.

After Nancy fell asleep, I could still hear the pounding surf. I put my book down and turned off the light. Flashes of lightening touched corners of the room. Thunder resounded in the distance.

Closing my eyes, I thought about persistence, a word we would have to put to use very soon. Persistence and determination to withstand time. Time from Nancy's surgery until her complete recovery. But, no. I mustn't think about that now, only about tomorrow. Tomorrow and the week ahead of us were ours.

Despite the storm, somehow I knew it was meant to be like this. Just the two of us, mother and daughter, together on our island. With a smile of anticipation I slid down between the cool sheets and closed my eyes. Tomorrow would come sooner that way.

CHAPTER THREE

Lost and Found

The next morning was a lazy one, a swim in the pool, a short walk along the beach. Time to unwind. We found it usually took a day or two to slow down to island pace. After lunch I set my typewriter on the balcony table and began to type. I was enjoying a sip of coffee when Nancy walked out onto the deck.

"Want to take another walk along the beach, mom?"

She grasped the redwood chair, pushed it across the wide boards, then plunked herself down. Over the railing we could see the surf still pounding the beach. There had been no let up in the intensity of the waves, but yesterday's summer thunderstorms had worked their way further north.

Nancy repeated her question, "Want to go?"

"No. Not now. It's near three and..."

"Mind if I go?"

I shook my head. The tide was on its way out and we both knew it was the best time for shelling. I felt like staying put. Each to her own had always been our way on the island. As I pecked out another few words, Nancy disappeared beyond the French doors.

Moments later she was back, dressed in her yellow bathing shorts and halter top, my new stovepipe sun hat perched unsteadily on her head. She carried a shirt for cover-up, remembering Dr. Keiser's warning not to get sunburned. She stood in the doorway looping the pink ties of my sun hat under her chin.

"Mind if I borrow it?"

I shook my head, smiling.

"Knew you wouldn't, mom."

She blew me a kiss and was off down the stairway. I saw her again on the beach path and watched her every movement. She reached the water's edge taking the whole distance in the quick, easy steps of a seventeen-year-old. Except for the slight hitch in her right hip, they were not the steps of a girl facing major spinal surgery. They were the steps of a young woman nearing maturity who has her whole wonderful life ahead of her. Nancy was both.

She stood there gazing southward toward the waves as they rose and fell on their sweep inland from the horizon. Then she turned right and walked westward, swinging her plastic shelling bag in her hand.

After she disappeared beyond the palms and pines lining the beach, I left the balcony long enough to refill my coffee cup from the steaming pot on the stove. When I returned, I set the cup down beside my typewriter, giving little thought to my papers and books strewn about. Unorganized as they appeared, they were a means of organization to me, a means of placing in true perspective all the things about me. For this, to me, was what writing was all about. I began to type. Words formed beneath my fingertips. There was a joy and detachment in doing so, as if I was exploring a world beyond the real that was even more real, more vivid. It had a depth and meaning and fulfillment that, when completed, brought me back closer in understanding of the actual world.

Time slipped away.

Suddenly I became aware of the moment. My coffee cup was empty. For the first time since starting to type I looked at my watch. Nearly six o'clock!

I stood up, stretched, and moved to the railing, rubbing the stiffness from my legs. The palms and sea grape cast long shadows on the beach path. Westward, toward the sinking sun, there was no yellow swimsuit in sight, no stovepipe hat, no firm young body swinging along. Eastward, there was hardly a soul on the beach. Grasping the railing, everything became unimportant except Nancy. She had been gone long enough for me to be uneasy and it was not like her to make me worry.

From the balcony to the beach took me, well, I don't know how long, because I literally transported myself down onto the sand. At the edge of the turning tide the foam washed over my feet and the sea looked like a giant overflowing basin. As it swept toward me I felt it was going to grasp me, pull me under and out.

What a silly, morbid thought! Everything had an explanation. The storms of the past few days explained the murky, churning water. My pleasure-seeking bit had momentarily gone askew. I'd better get it back into working order promptly. There would be plenty of time for seriousness in the months to come.

Walking westward as Nancy had done, I turned to look eastward just in case she had retraced her steps and gone toward the lighthouse. But I was sure she hadn't. Once on a definite course she rarely turned back. Almost eighteen years had shown me her dogged determination, so much like her father's.

As I continued, each sheller nodded at my passing, a custom on the island. Strangers, yet friends. A kinship rarely found on any city street. A kinship brought about by the sea. Just a simple smile, a nod and "hi." Then a passing on. One after the other, the shellers were heading back. I kept going, scanning the beach for a familiar figure, but still not seeing her.

When the sun dropped behind a bank of dark clouds, the Gulf took on that eerie but beautiful gray-green shade of water just before a storm. There were no storms in sight, though. The sky was a deep blue with only a scattering of clouds and the dark bank along the horizon to the west.

As I walked on, the lap edge of each wave sent the sand squishing between my toes, then washed them clean with the next wave. I had passed everyone in sight. Suddenly I saw a speck on the horizon. I kept looking ahead at the speck, then down to my feet. Ahead and down. Only then did I notice the hundreds of broken and crushed shells. Conchs. Turkey Wings. Scallops. Cones. Were they all here on the lesser-traveled end of the beach?

I began to hum as I continued my trek. The speck on the horizon became a toothpick silhouette. It took form and moved toward me. I waved. No wave back. I began to run. I dug my toes into the grains of sand beneath my feet and scattered them as I ran, trying not to land on any broken shells.

I ran until my heart beat hard and the beat rose up into my throat. My breathing came in gulps. My legs gave out on a stretch of beach where the pines and palms parted long enough to expose a weather-beaten house, shuttered and still, its gables and chimneys giving it a Gothic air. I started walking at a faster pace to hurry by.

Ahead, the toothpick silhouette took life. I recognized the hitch in the quick step. Pink ribbons attached to the sun hat blew in the south breeze. We both waved at the same time and ran toward each other. I still don't know where my legs regained the strength, but they moved me forward until we met.

I touched her arm, pink from her afternoon on the beach. I wanted to spank her and gather her in my arms all at once. I did neither.

"Where have you been?" I scolded. "You've been gone so long. Why did you walk so far?" All at once the questions came tumbling out.

"I just felt like walking," she answered.

It was as simple as that. Most seventeen-year-olds learned to cope with motherly concern by developing a pseudo-blasé defense. But, underneath it all, there was thankfulness for the concern.

Admit it?

Never. Not in so many words. It was sort of playing ball with feelings, throwing them back and forth. All the while, inside the ball, under the covering of worldly sophistication, lay the most important ingredient in human relationships, that of caring deeply.

Now the moment of ball throwing was over and we were two adults, talking.

"I'm sorry if I worried you. I really didn't mean to."

"It's all right, as long as you're all right," I said and turned to fall in step beside her.

Perhaps she needed the walk, time alone to sort out her thoughts. The surgery, the casts. Those were not easy things to accept. Even though her dad and I would be right there beside her all the way, the test was going to be within herself.

"Did you find any good shells?"

"A few."

She opened her shell bag, letting me take a look. We headed back following the edge of the water, our heads bent, still searching for shells. Maybe we'd find a lacy murex or olive shell worth picking up.

For a long distance the quiet was only broken by the rise and fall of the surf, reaching into us, closer, closer. Forward, then back. Forward, then back.

Finally, Nancy spoke. "I don't ever remember the sea this rough before. Do you? And another thing, mom. Remember how the egrets and sandpipers would run ahead of us, then take off and land further up the beach? I've seen hardly any."

I nodded. She was right. Nowhere around us were there any birds or whole shells. There was nothing except the sea, the sand and the two of us walking together. A cold shiver crossed my shoulders and goose bumps stood out on my arms. Was I letting my emotions point to negative things that didn't exist? Or, if they did, existed naturally and rightfully?

Nancy moved ahead of me and walked up towards the high tide line, all the while her head bent in search of another shell. I continued on by the water's edge. We were well on our way back to the apartment when she dropped to her knees.

"MOM! Quick!"

I caught up to her and looked down at what she had found. There in the sand, amidst broken and crushed shells, lay two Angel Wings, both about five inches long. I knelt beside her and we each picked one up. Gently we rubbed our fingers over the edges, ridges and inside. We had always heard they were a treasure in pairs. That ours were two left Angel Wings made no difference.

"They're beautiful!" Nancy said in a hushed whisper, rubbing hers against her cheek.

I stared at the one in my hand and felt its firm strength despite its fragility. "They are beautiful! And they do resemble an Angel's Wing! See here? This is the hinge that must have joined to an Angel's back."

"Oh, come on, mom!" Nancy laughed and put her shell beside mine as we knelt in the sand together.

Sudden warmth touched us. We both turned back

toward the west to see that the sun had reached a rim of blue sky just above the horizon, between the sea and the bank of dark clouds. A golden glow touched the clouds, tinted the sea, the sand and embraced the two of us.

CHAPTER FOUR

Storing Memories

On our second morning we awoke early. I opened the French doors to our balcony and stepped out into a New World. Morning sunshine threw sparkling strands of silver across the Gulf. Waves rolled in, softly lapping the shore. I took in a deep breath of fresh air. Delicious! Nancy felt it too. She joined me on the balcony and stretched her arms out wide.

"Mmm! What a day!"

We both leaned forward over the balcony railing. Several pelicans bobbed in the gentle swells just offshore. Our sandpipers were back too, dancing their carousel, twittering and turning like funny little people. Standing there I felt the security of nature's seclusion.

"I'll fix breakfast, mom."

Nancy straightened to her full five-foot-eight inches. Her legs and feet were bare, her baby doll pajamas hugging her hips high on the right side. She made the familiar gesture of pulling them down even with the left side, both of us knowing they would only hitch up again.

"Want bacon and eggs?"

"Sounds fine," I answered, following her as far as the low bookcase divider in the apartment. There I picked up the two Angel Wings and carried them back to the balcony. I could study them better in the sunlight. With one in each hand I sat down on a porch chair. I closed my eyes for a few moments, letting the sounds of the sea envelope me.

The aroma of sizzling bacon and perking coffee brought me back to the balcony and the soft rhythm of the surf. Placing the two Angel Wings on the table in front of me, I counted down from the hinge point of one. Twenty-eight ribs flowed out fanlike, covering the whole shell from blunt shoulder to bottom. Twenty-eight ribs with dips like little valleys in between.

Both must be the same I thought. Out of curiosity, I counted the second. Twenty-nine ribs! Surely my eyes were failing me or my counting was off. I counted again. Twenty-nine. I recounted the first shell. Twenty-eight. Odd...

Near the eighth and ninth rib on one was a tiny hole I hadn't noticed before. Strange how many things escape us when we don't look closely enough. I checked the number of ribs again. Twenty-eight and twenty-nine. Why? I knew little about Angel Wings, only what I had read in our shell book. Was the difference due to age? Or was it an imperfection? Without comparison each looked perfect.

Is perfection just a relative condition?

Nancy's spine was imperfect. The S shape had a 50-degree thoracic curve and a 70-degree lumbar curve. Severe idiopathic scoliosis, Dr. Keiser at Miami's Variety Children's Hospital had termed it.

I was turning the Angel Wings over in my hands when Nancy broke my thought pattern.

"Almost ready!" She called from the kitchenette.

"Great! I'm starved!"

I put the Angel Wings down as she came out with the breakfast trays. Frosty orange juice, bacon cooked just right, eggs, toast and steaming cups of coffee.

"Now there's a meal fit for a beachcomber."

"Right, mom."

Nancy sat beside me, raising her juice glass. "Here's to the best shelling ever."

"I'll drink to that!" I said.

And we did.

That week we were like two hungry pelicans. We often watched them swoop down and pluck fish out of the sea. Seven days were all we had to store up against the months to come. We walked the beach, drifted in the edge-tide and swam in the pool. As I lay in the sun, Nancy would dive in and swim the length of the pool underwater. Slim, quick, seemingly strong, her performance made it hard to believe she needed anything done to her back.

"Hey, mom! Watch!"

I took my sunglasses off and sat up in the chaise.

Nancy threw a penny into the pool. It swirled and bubbled to the bottom. Then straight down she dove, picked up the penny and rose to the surface. With a shake of her head, she called to me.

"How about that, mom? You want to try it?"

"Me? Never! You're the mermaid. I'm the sun-dowser!"

We shared a closeness that week, a closeness without suffocation. An understanding needing few words. Our thoughts ran along similar lines, yet never collided. She was at the breaking away age, but for the next year she would be completely dependent upon her father and me. After that she would be on her own and we would let her go. That was as it should be.

Each day after finding the Angel Wings we picked them up and turned them over in curiosity. There was a truth about them that we never expressed in exact words. They were to become more precious to us than all the other shells we collected. At a shell shop on the island we bought a large black shell box with a glass cover. After cleaning the best shells, Nancy arranged them with the Angel Wings taking center stage.

Each morning we opened the French doors to the balcony, breathed in the salty sea air and listened to the surf. We ate breakfast and lunch in privacy there. We enjoyed supper and sat in the twilight until the mosquitoes drove us in for the night. Each evening I sat and read while Nancy picked over the new additions to her shell collection. Each night we slept a good, deep sleep.

Seven days, seven nights, a well of memories, endless words, many shells, dozens of walks by the sea with the blue of the sky and the gold of the sun reaching down, filling us. On our last night we stood on the balcony looking out at a sliver of moon in a deep black sky.

"Mom, a year from now, when it's all over and I'm out of the casts, let's come back. Do you think we can?"

I looked over at my daughter standing beside me. Still part child, yet almost woman. Eighteen was a wonderful age. The time of bewilderment was slowly passing and the time of true discovery and piecing together of life was beginning in earnest. Inwardly, I knew we could never come back to this moment. Once we turned from the balcony only the memory would remain.

"We can try," I said, hugging her tight.

The next day we left our island. We drove back over the causeway and bridge, crossing the three miles of water, deep and swirling on both sides.

Forward.

There is a kind of excitement in facing life's intensities. Birth. Love. War. Storms. Obstacles. Trials.

"It will be an adventure," I had said a month before. "Let's treat the next year in just that way."

"Sure, mom," Nancy had replied.

I gazed at her light brown hair tied back into two pigtails, her face fresh, young and eager for life. At almost eighteen the biggest tragedy for her, I thought, was not starting college with all her friends. Could she accept the near total immobility for the next six months? Months in which she would be in casts from neck to hips? Then how many more months wearing a brace? What about after that? Would she be able to go back to the vibrant living she now had?

We reached the mainland and tollbooth at Punta Rassa. Both of us turned and looked back across the blue waters to the Sanibel shoreline. Near Bailey's General Store, the ancient mail-dock was scarcely visible. Even though I couldn't see them, I knew our pelicans perched there on the pilings. We had always called them the official greeters to the island. We would miss them.

We turned forward again. Nancy pressed her foot on the accelerator, her slender fingers sure on the steering wheel. Sure in a way I wished I could be. Leaving our island was always hard on us. For a long time we were silent, thinking thoughts we never revealed to each other.

CHAPTER FIVE

Surgery is Over

I felt a hand on my arm.

"Hi, sleepy head," Fred said in his gentle voice.

I looked up at him, rubbing my eyes. "Was I asleep?"

Fred nodded. "You needed the nap. What were you dreaming about?"

I smiled. "Sanibel. And how hard it was to leave the island."

All around me I heard the busy sounds of Taylor Pavilion.

"Have we had any more news?"

Fred shook his head no. "It's nearly eleven. Why don't we take the doctor's advice and get some lunch. He said he would find us when surgery is done."

As we walked toward the cafeteria we could smell the aroma of food cooking. It all smelled so good, but I wondered if I could eat any lunch. Fred chose a table for four and I sat while he went to fill our trays. He returned with two plates of steaming food and set one down in front of me.

"Try some," he said.

I picked up my fork and took a mouthful, finding it did taste delicious. We noticed a young couple looking around for a place to sit and asked them to join us. We exchanged first names. They told us about their very ill child.

Fred said, "I am so sorry. We all must pray for our children."

Sadly the young mother replied, "Yes. All we can do now is pray."

As we looked around we saw parents reaching out to other parents. They, as we, knew what heartache was. Each was trying to give the other encouragement. Slowly, two by two, couples finished eating. I could hear chairs being pushed back and bits of conversation.

"God bless you. We shall pray for your child too."

We returned to Taylor Pavilion for the final wait. Shortly after noon, we heard the news we had been waiting for. Dr. Keiser approached us.

"Mr. and Mrs. Webster? It's all over. Everything went as planned. Your daughter is doing fine."

"Thank you doctor." I could find no other words. This wonderful human being, this skilled surgeon had given Nancy hope for the future and all I could say was thank you. And thanks to God there was help for her scoliosis. Thanks to God for Dr. Keiser who made it happen.

In looking back, I realized no other words were necessary. I'm sure he must have sensed our relief and gratitude. After he left us, I sat down. My knees were unsteady like those of a child beginning to walk. Yet I wanted to run up and down the corridor and shout, "It's all over! It's all over!" Instead I sat with my palms over my cheeks, trying to hold back the onrushing inside of me. My eyes were moist and I blinked the tears away as I watched another doctor approach us.

"Hello. Are you the Websters?"

Fred nodded.

"I assisted Dr. Keiser. He did a beautiful job. Your daughter is really straight now. She'll progress rapidly. She has the healthiest bones of any child we've seen."

Healthy bones? Of course. All the milk we'd been prodding her to drink for years. Images flashed through my mind. I could see an endless line of milk bottles. As each one was emptied, it fell over like a domino. But if her bones were exceptionally healthy, then why the curvature? Would we ever know?

The doctor continued, "And just think. Your daughter is almost three inches taller." He smiled, wished us well and went on his way.

My mouth fell open. Fred looked at me and laughed. After a moment, it sank in. Why, of course. A straight line was the shortest distance between two points. Basic geometry. Thus, any curve when straightened would cover a greater distance. It never occurred to me to apply the rule to Nancy. But three inches?

"Come on," Fred said. "We won't be able to see Nancy for some time. So, while you're thinking that one over, let's go get another cup of coffee and some dessert. Now that our daughter is taller than you are, you're going to need all that extra nourishment to keep her in line."

As we sat again in the cafeteria, we talked about all the people who had donated blood in Nancy's name. Family, friends, neighbors, men who worked with Fred and had never even met Nancy. Nine in all gave a pint of their blood to be held in reserve at the blood bank. Many others offered.

How could we possibly say thank you for such a gift? We knew we couldn't. There were no words to express such gratitude. We could only thank God for the goodness of man. Times like these bring out the kindness we are all capable of offering. They reconfirm our faith that life is not futile. There is a reason for our existence, a purpose for our lives.

It was nearly four-thirty before Nancy returned from the recovery room. Fred and I were sitting in the same small waiting room in Taylor Pavilion when she was wheeled back through the swinging doors with a pint of blood still dripping into her veins. A nurse held the bottle of plasma high as she walked alongside the procession.

Realizing the seriousness of every move, Fred and I stayed out of the way, but craned our necks to see our daughter. Nancy's eyes were closed and her face mirrored the sweet innocence of the child she had been; the child she would always be to us.

Steady hands moved her stretcher along slowly and with obvious care. Fred and I followed and waited until the nurses had settled her in bed. We had hired special nurses who would attend to Nancy in shifts during the first 24 critical hours after surgery.

Critical hours? From now on, until her cast was applied, every hour was critical. Any wrong move or sudden jerk could dislodge the steel rods anchored inside her back and she would end up in surgery again.

When one of the nurses motioned us to come in, Fred and I walked quietly to Nancy's side. Her eyes fluttered and opened. She smiled and closed them. I placed my fingertips on her forehead and trailed them down, cupping her cheek with my palm.

Her eyes fluttered open a second time. "Hi, mom. Hi, dad."

Her words were slow and slurred, but they were all we wanted to hear. We stepped back so the nurse could attend to her without any interference. Nancy needed rest and constant care, the kind our unskilled hands and unspecialized knowledge could not provide. In a way, right now, we were outside her life. We could only be onlookers.

As we sat in silence, I noticed Nancy's bed had been turned around. Her feet were at the head and her head at the foot. The crank for raising and lowering the bed had been removed as well. One of the aides explained that all "rod patients" were turned head to foot as an extra precaution. And removal of the elevating crank eliminated the chance of anyone accidentally raising the bed. She would also be kept on her side, propped with pillows fore and aft to keep her spine absolutely straight and immobile.

Nurses came and went. An intravenous bottle replaced the last bottle of plasma. Frequent checks were made and our special nurse never left Nancy's side. At seven that evening, she came over and placed her hand on my shoulder. "I know how you feel. You want to stay. But Nancy hardly knows you're here. She's going to be all right. You're both tired. Why don't you go home and get some rest?"

She was right. We were tired. Achingly tired. But so hopeful and so relieved. We took her advice and headed home.

CHAPTER SIX

Thirteen Days

We left Nancy in her hospital bed by the window. We had been advised to go home and get some rest, but I knew I wouldn't be able to. How could I? My dear child was alone in a hospital room not able to talk, or even know that she was alone.

Fred, restless himself, said, "You'd better get some rest. You'll be wearing yourself out." He worried about my worrying. I knew he missed our girl as much as I did.

I slept in Nancy's room that first night. The hospital might call saying she needed me. I didn't trust myself to hear the phone in the kitchen. And, although the nurse had assured us there would be no reason to call, I felt better resting next to Nancy's white princess phone with its illuminated dial. It was like a lifeline to the hospital and the room where she lay.

During the next four days Nancy was kept sedated with painkillers. Each morning I drove the 25 miles to the hospital and stayed until it was time to go home and fix Fred's supper. Then we both returned to sit by her side until visiting hours were over. Nancy was groggy; she would say a few words and then drop off to sleep again.

We would whisper, "Remember the Angel Wings." We hoped, somehow, she could hear us.

Dr. Keiser came in each day, both to check on Nancy and to reassure me of her progress. His miracle hands had accomplished straightening her spine and his gentle voice calmed my fears. He explained that, with the Harrington Rod, he had been able to correct her spinal curve to10-degrees thoracic / 25-degrees lumbar, increasing her height by over two inches.

He had used calf bone for the fusion rather than taking Nancy's own bone, saving her from additional surgery and a scar on her leg. He explained that calf bone was a new method developed by Squibb and had been approved by the Food and Drug Administration in early January 1965. Nancy was a pioneer of sorts in its use.

Years later we found out that the experimentation with calf bone was short lived. Doctors discovered it did not have the strength, nor fuse as well as the patient's own bone. But, to Nancy, not having a scar on her leg was a relief.

Nurses came in and log-rolled Nancy every two hours. Her turning from one side to the other was a planned procedure involving teamwork. Two nurses and Nancy. Lying on a draw sheet and with a nurse on each side of the bed, she was pulled gently toward the edge she faced.

Then came the commands, "Knees up. Elbows bent. Come on honey. Now roll. One. Two. Three."

By the count of three, the nurses had rolled her like a log onto her back and over to the other side. Even though sedated, she would moan, then settle down. The nurses would fluff her pillows and tuck them fore and aft again, giving her a pat of encouragement, "Good girl."

One evening Fred and I brought tiny tea roses. Nancy winced as she tried to reach out to touch them. I pushed them within easy reach. "Nice, mom. Nice, dad." Then she closed her eyes again.

A little later she awoke, looked up at me and asked, "Mom? How tall am I now?"

I smiled and answered, "You're two and a half inches taller, dear."

"Wow..." She closed her eyes and went back to sleep.

Friends and family visited, tried to make conversation, then left, realizing it would be awhile before Nancy could respond fully. Flowers arrived, filling the table and windowsill. More cards came each day. How could I possibly thank everyone for their prayers, kindness and generosity?

By the fifth day the little tea roses had wilted. In contrast, Nancy came to life. She was aware now of the goings on and of the discomfort, but she didn't want any more drugs. She'd had enough floating and wanted back in the real world. That was were the living was. With the discontinuance of the drugs, her eyes cleared and she looked directly at me.

"What day is it?"

"Tuesday." I got up out of the chair and went to her.

"Tuesday? Where did Friday, Saturday, Sunday and Monday go?"

"They went whoosh, right out that door. Just as these flowers will have to."

"I remember only a little. I remember you and dad standing beside me. Then voices. And Stephanie. And... It's a jumble."

"Of course it is right now, but you'll unscramble it.

Later that afternoon, Stephanie bounced in with her "Hiya kid!" greeting. She sat by Nancy's side holding her hand, talking gently to her, thinking it better not to try and make her laugh just yet.

The next morning before I started off to the hospital, I walked around the yard, looking at our shrubs and plants. For days I hadn't had a chance to see them, nor had I cared. As I came to our gardenia bush I stopped. May was their month for blooming and they had bloomed profusely. This was July. I looked at the bush, unbelieving. There were five gardenia blooms and more ready to burst open. I picked the five open blooms, took them into the house and placed them in a bowl, careful not to touch the white petals.

An hour later at the hospital I put them on the table beside Nancy.

"Oh, mom! Gardenias!" She hesitated. "I thought they were finished blooming for this year!"

"So did I."

She looked at me, then back at the bowl. I wondered if she was thinking the same as me. How much the white petals resembled the whiteness of the two Angel Wing shells.

"They're pretty, mom."

Suddenly I remembered back years before to a pasture and a little girl of three who had said the same thing about dandelions. I swallowed hard and answered as I had then, "Yes, darling. Very pretty."

The staff took excellent care of Nancy. Mabel, a nurse's aide, was assigned to Nancy. Mabel, big, strong and jolly, had the gentle caress of an angel as she smoothed back Nancy's hair with her dimpled black hands. She was the nurses' second wind and knew the routine of the "rod patients" from beginning to end. Her adopted "children" were her legion, her love and patience were endless, her concern genuine, and her experience faultless. She wasn't about to have any of her little ones end up back in surgery. Her reward was in the tone of voice the children used when they called out, "Mabel! Mabel! I need you!"

Nancy began the slow process of beginning to eat again. Liquids at first, then more solid foods. I kept hearing the same phrase repeated over and over, *"she can't go home until she has had a movement."* How could such a simple process become so important?

I believe Nancy fell in love with Dr. Keiser. Or, perhaps it was simply hero worship. For making her straight, he was almost a God in her eyes. When he came in, checked her incision and said, "Ahumm," she would weigh his every word. She wanted to do everything he advised, to be his star patient and he made her feel as though she was. Although quick and clinical with the nurses and staff, he was tender, warm and understanding with the children.

Nancy planned for the next year to go as scheduled with no setbacks. Then there would be college, horseback riding, boys. The joy of living. She laid still when told to, rolled when instructed, ate, drank and did everything to make sure her chart had all the correct entries.

Steph always entered Nancy's room with her bouncing step, her smiling eyes and cheery, "Hiya kid!" greeting. Some days she knew Nan didn't feel up to it. Steph would touch her arm and say, "Don't feel so great? I know. So don't talk." What little Stephanie said was in soft tones. A word or two about the kids and goings on. I blessed her for knowing when to leave.

And her other friends did too. Another of Nancy's friends, Pam, came to visit often. Pam knew what it was all about having been through the surgery the previous year. A sweet pain filled me as I witnessed the loyalty young people could have for one another; the insight we often didn't give them credit for.

Each day I brought freshly cut gardenias from our

own backyard bush. The bush continued to bloom and did so for an exceptionally long time that year. Nancy would hold the white flowers, taking in their delightful smell and tell me of the happenings from the previous night. Sleeping was difficult for her. She would wake up to strange noises and children screaming.

The bed next to her was eventually filled. Nancy's roommate was younger than she and cried constantly. Whether from pain or loneliness, I was never quite sure. She would thrash her arms and legs, trying to move herself until the pain stopped her and the nurses came in to hold her and talk to her. She tried everyone's patience. She'd gone through the spinal fusion like Nancy, but was not accepting it. By not doing so, she took the chance of ending right back at the beginning. We had heard of more than one case that had to go back in for more long hours of surgery. Nancy lay there listening, trying to console her, but to no use.

I was puzzled that she rarely had visitors. Each day I made it a point to stop by her bed to try to cheer her up, but it didn't seem to help. Her screams became so disruptive that she was eventually moved into a private room. But even with Nancy's door closed tight, we still heard the remnants of her cries and for weeks afterward they remained in our minds, to haunt us and make us wonder how she had come out of it all.

On the twelfth day Dr. Keiser said Nancy was ready for her cast. Her incision had healed without any infection. She was impatient and ready long before the aides wheeled a stretcher into her room. That morning my fear was of my own reaction to seeing her in a cast from neck to hips. How would I take it?

"I wonder what it's like," she mused.

"I don't know," I answered. "But don't you forget a thing. I want to hear all about it." I pretended nonchalance as I kissed her.

Minutes later, as her stretcher rolled out of the room and down the hall, Nancy called back, "I'll take notes, mom!" She tapped her head, then blew me a kiss.

This time I waited alone. I walked up and down the hall for a while, then came back to Nancy's room and sat in silence by her empty bed. I gazed out the window beyond the parking lot to several palms swaying on the lawn. July breezes rustled the fronds and the sun beat down. Some of the sun's heat entered the window and touched me. The warmth of it began to penetrate my heart. It would be all right. What was I afraid of? Hadn't I been waiting anxiously for her to be put in the protective cast? It would be all right.

I wasn't prepared, though, when the stretcher rolled into the room with Nancy lying stiff and straight.

"Hi, mom! Here I am!" Nancy said as the aides transferred her from the stretcher to the bed.

"Hi." I turned so she wouldn't see me dabbing at the corner of my eyes. It must have been the sun that made them water. Then I went to her. From the cast top to her chin was a metal bar with a chin rest. In the back was another metal bar with a head rest.

"How do you like it?" Nancy threw off the blanket, revealing a formal gown of Plaster of Paris.

"Quite original, I'd say."

"Look at all the space for signatures!"

All I could think of was what could I whip up for fashionable attire for the next three months.

Nancy began to tell me about her experience. She had been taken downstairs for x-rays and then to the cast room, or "torture room" as some of the children called it.

"It was really something," she went on. "They put me on this thing. Kind of like a bed frame. They called it a Stryker frame. I sort of hung there and I was scared of falling through, but there were plenty of people holding on to me. Then they put this long body stocking on me, then lots of cotton, and then they wound me round and round with gauze. And, know what?"

"No. What?"

"The gauze was soaked in hot Plaster of Paris. I mean, HOT! I actually steamed! Then, after the plaster started drying they attached these metal bars to the front and back so I have a place to rest my chin and my head."

I touched the cast. It still felt moist. "Cover up," I said. "You don't want pneumonia."

"I'm not worried about that." Nancy looked straight

at me as I smoothed the covers over her.

"What then?" I asked.

"Oh, nothing. I guess it's silly. But what if I got appendicitis while I was in this thing?"

"Now you really are being silly," I said. "Appendicitis?"

"Sure, mom. It could happen you know."

Yes, it could happen. She could have appendicitis while in the cast. Why worry about it, though? Too many other things could happen too. We would just take the days one at a time.

The first twelve days were gone. We had survived them. Maybe the rest wouldn't be so bad after all. Besides, tomorrow was July 20th, a very special day.

Nancy's eighteenth birthday!

When Mabel came in to roll Nancy over, she worked gently. "How's that, lamb?"

"Fine." Nancy lay facing the window and me, now safely confined in the armor that was to be her dress for the next 84 days.

Mabel smoothed the covers over her. "Keep warm, baby."

"I will." Suddenly she burst out. "Oh, my gosh!"

"What? Anything wrong?" Mabel leaned over to check.

"No..." Nancy hesitated, then reconsidered. "Yes. Tomorrow's my birthday. My EIGHTEENTH birthday! When will Dr. Keiser be in? I've just GOT to see him!"

"In a while. Don' you worry none." Mabel gave Nancy a pat on the arm. As she hurried out she turned back for a moment. "Your eighteenth birthday, eh? Well, fancy that."

It wasn't long before Dr. Keiser came in. He went through his usual routine. His words with nurses. Low words I probably wouldn't have understood anyway. Then he checked Nancy's cast and asked some questions. With the serious business out of the way he always took time to be the children's friend as well as their doctor.

"How are you doing?" he asked.

"Great," Nancy answered. She bit the corner of her lip and her voice was shaky as she spoke. "Do you think I could go home tomorrow?"

"Tomorrow?" Why tomorrow? Aren't you happy here with us?"

"Yes. Well, I guess. But tomorrow." She looked up at him with the same expression she had used on her father and me so many times. "Tomorrow is my birthday."

"Your birthday?" Dr. Keiser readjusted his glasses on his nose. "Your birthday? Well." He placed his finger on his chin as if in deep thought. "How old will you be? Sixteen?"

"Dr. Keiser! You know I'm going to be eighteen!"

"Hmm. Eighteen. And you want to go home because tomorrow is your birthday."

The lines on his forehead deepened.

"Oh, Dr. Keiser, can I? Can I, please? I'll do anything you say. Please!"

He looked over at me. In his eyes I could see his understanding and compassion.

"We want to do what you think is best," I said.

Nancy's eyes were filling with tears. He took her hand in his.

"An eighteenth birthday is pretty important, isn't it?"

Nancy nodded.

He cleared his throat. "I think it can be arranged."

"Oh, thank you doctor. Thank you!" Nancy looked up at him, not even seeming to care that two big tears had rolled down her cheeks.

CHAPTER SEVEN

Coming Home

An eighteenth birthday? What a time for celebration! And celebrate we would. On the way home from the hospital, I stopped by the bakery and ordered a big square birthday cake. There would have to be punch and ice cream too. My mind whirled with the thought. Nancy's coming home tomorrow!

Her friends all wanted to be there. Once again our home would burst with laughter. Oh, how good that would be after her seemingly endless thirteen days in the hospital. But, first, we had to get Nancy home.

Finally, the morning of July twentieth arrived. I could scarcely contain my excitement. We borrowed my friend Mac's station wagon and with Stephanie's Aunt Maud sitting beside me, we started out for Variety Children's Hospital. In the back lay the stretcher Fred had made from a sheet of plywood. He had cut and smoothed the edges and made two handle holes on each end for carrying. We had added a mattress and several blankets and pillows. Fred and Steph's Uncle Don were at home ready to meet us when we returned with our precious cargo.

A half-hour later at the hospital I went through the usual routine of patient release, looking over papers, checking insurance records and signing releases. Finally I was given the okay.

Up in Taylor Pavilion other things were happening. When I arrived at the nursing station there was a gathering of on duty nurses with Mabel right in the middle of it all. On the counter sat a birthday cake with eighteen candles.

"Get 'em all lit!" Mabel said as she and the head nurse lit all eighteen wicks. At that moment Mabel was chief of staff and had everything under control. I watched as she picked up the cake and turned towards Nancy's room. We all followed and began to sing:

"Happy birthday, dear Nancy,
Happy birthday to you!"

I felt a tightness inside me; an onrushing of warmth as Mabel carefully set the cake down beside Nancy's bed.

"There, darlin'," she said. "Blow 'em all out an' yu'll surely get your wish. Here, mama..." Mabel pulled me through the group of nurses and crowd of children to Nancy's side. "Yur mama has to be here too, girl!"

Nancy looked up at me. "Gee. Hi, mom!" I touched her arm and bent down to kiss her forehead.

Mabel, still beside me said, "There darlin'. Go ahead. Blow."

The candles on Nancy's cake glimmered in the crowded hospital room. Nancy blew and blew until every candle was out. Her breath must have been completely gone, but somehow I knew she would do it.

"Did you wish?" Mabel asked.

"Yes." Nancy looked up at the many faces around her bed. "I wished a good one."

"It'll come true then." Mabel helped Nancy cut the first piece, then cut the rest for the children. Gleefully each child reached for a piece of the gooey, rich cake and yelled to Nancy, "Good luck!"

Several of the children lingered by her bedside. One little girl asked, "You're really going home?"

"You better believe it!" Nancy giggled as she finished eating her piece of cake.

"That's neat!" she said.

Each child took turns autographing Nan's cast. Then, calling back their good-byes, they shuffled out and down the hall, singing all the way.

While we waited for the gurney, I packed up all her cards and decided which flower bouquets to take home, leaving the rest for the nurses to distribute among the other children's rooms. Two orderlies came into the room, transferring Nancy onto a hospital gurney. We were finally ready to leave.

Nancy's face beamed as hospital personnel wheeled the gurney to the station wagon where Maud was standing by. They carefully transferred her from the gurney to the stretcher Fred had made, slid it carefully into the back and then surrounded her with all the extra blankets and pillows we had brought. Once Nancy was settled we started our journey home. The drive seemed endless. My stomach was queasy and my hands gripped the wheel so tightly my knuckles turned white. To add to my jitters we encountered one of our typical summer afternoon thunderstorms. I was conscious of beating rain, slick roads and every car around me.

By the time we reached our driveway the storm had passed, but the sidewalks were still wet and the grass was full of sparkling dew. Fred and Don were waiting for us.

"Thank God. You're home safe!" Fred gave me a big hug as he helped me out of the car.

Fred got in and backed the car up on the front lawn and as close to the front door as possible.

At that moment our neighbor, Mel, came over from his home across the street, smiling. "Need some help?"

The three men carefully slid the wooden stretcher to the edge of the back of the station wagon. Fred and Don each held one corner while Mel lifted the end of the stretcher. They slowly made their way to the front door, but found they couldn't fit the stretcher and themselves through the opening at the same time. They had to lay the stretcher down and slide it into the house, then get their hands under the bottom, lift it and turn the corner down the hall leading to Nancy's room. They carefully shifted her from the stretcher onto her bed, then slid the heavy wood under her bed.

"I'm home! I can't believe I'm home! Oh, this is the most beautiful house in the whole world!" Her excitement was contagious.

What she didn't know was that there was going to be a party. After all she had gone through we wanted to tell her slowly. Suddenly we heard voices at our front door. The party had already started. I knew now I had no way of easing her into it.

Her dear friends, Jill and Pam, were among the first to arrive, followed by many of her classmates and Sunday school class members. Laughter and young voices filled our home from the front steps, through the house to Nancy's room and out to the back patio.

"Nancy's home! Nancy's home!"

Then I heard the most familiar voice of all. Stephanie arrived with her "Hiya kid!" greeting. She ran down the hall towards Nancy's room, arms outstretched. Sisters? They could not have been more like sisters than if they had been born twins.

Each friend passing through Nancy's bedroom brought gifts, cards, thoughts, little things meaning so much, especially gentle hugs and smiles. There was paper strewn all over the bed and floor, laughter and giggles, young people back and forth to the dining room table for cake and ice-cream and punch. It was wild and noisy and wonderful. It turned out to be an evening not be forgotten.

I could see the love and respect each friend had for Nancy. She was a youngster who tried never to let anyone see her cry. That night I saw the tears that filled her eyes, as if to say, "I love you all." I am sure they all loved her back. I turned away, my own eyes brimming, my heart so full I thought it might burst.

Nancy was home!

Steph stayed right by Nancy's side the whole evening, hovering over her, making sure she was okay. Toward the end of the party she came to me and said she thought Nan was tired and not feeling well. When I went into check on Nancy, she looked pale and I assumed she was exhausted from the excitement of her homecoming and all her friends gathered around. We quietly shuffled the last of her friends out the door and I settled Nancy in for her first night at home.

That first night, not unlike her first night home as a baby, I felt an overwhelming uneasiness of my job and what lay ahead. Particularly the knowledge Nancy was powerless to move from one spot to another without help. During the previous spring, Fred had installed small air-conditioners in our bedroom and in Nancy's. That meant that both our door and hers remained closed and I was afraid I would not be able to hear her if she needed me.

"What are you doing, mom?" Nancy asked as I picked up a chair and placed its back against the edge of her bed. When I set a second one on the other side, she almost flipped on her own. "For Pete sakes, mom, I'm not a baby. I won't fall out."

The mother instinct in me felt better knowing the chairs were there, but I slept barely a wink that night. I kept imagining sounds, a chair moving, a thump, a call, but whenever I went to check, she lay on her side, eyes closed tight, just as I had left her. The sleep of the young, the sleep of the relaxed.

Our first crisis did come the next morning. Nancy, now eighteen, found it both difficult and embarrassing that I would have to sponge bathe her and attend to her bedpans. She didn't seem to mind the fact that the nurses had attended to her, but for her mother to do the same was unthinkable.

That first morning, in tears, she refused her bath. I knew I would have to convince her that this was how it was going to be and if I didn't do it today we would have a struggle every morning. I gently started washing her face, talking about something mundane, something to fill the quiet in the room. I moved on to her arms, her legs, leaving the rest for last. I covered her with towels and kept her as private as I possibly could. She closed her eyes and gritted her teeth, but I finished and I knew she must feel better. She finally relaxed her clenched teeth and grudgingly gave me a smile. Each day after that became a little easier; she more relaxed, me more confident in keeping her dignity.

We had survived our first crisis, but I expected there would be many more to follow.

Fred's words echoed in my mind, "Honey, you don't realize how much there is ahead of you to do. I hope this will not be too much for you to handle."

And my response? "It doesn't matter. She is my daughter. How could I do any less?"

Two nights later, in the wee hours of the morning, Nancy called out to me, "Mom! Mom! My stomach hurts really bad!"

I instantly realized my fears of not hearing her if she called out had been unfounded. I rushed into her room and turned on her bedside lamp. Her breathing was labored as she groaned in pain. She was pale, not just pale from the hospital stay, but a sick pale.

Where don't you feel good?" I asked.

"Ohh, right here." She tried to find the spot on her stomach. "All over."

I touched her cold clammy hands.

"Oh, mom. The cast. It's pressing where my stomach aches. Please, do something!"

She began to roll her head from side to side in distress. Distress or pain, I wondered and perhaps did a foolish thing. I reached for the Alka-Seltzer bottle and made her down a small dose. Moments later she was writhing in pain, beads of sweat standing out on her face and arms.

Within seconds I was on the phone to my friend, Mac. She was at our door in less than five minutes, still is her pajamas and housecoat. She hurried down the hall to Nancy's room, sat on the bed and took Nan's wrist between her thumb and four fingers. She felt her forehead, all the while gazing at her watch. She counted Nancy's breathing.

"What's wrong?" I asked.

She ignored my question. Not out of rudeness, but out of preoccupation with other matters. She began questioning Nancy, all the while still holding her wrist between her thumb and four fingers, every few moments rechecking her watch.

"What did you eat today?" she asked.

"Ohh..." Nancy's voice trailed off.

Mac asked again, "Nan? What did you have for dinner?"

"Mom fixed steak and veggies and I had some milk and fruit."

"Anything else?"

"Well. Yes. Steph and I finished a bag of potato chips. Ahh..."

Mac reached for the Kleenex box and dabbed Nancy's forehead and arms.

"Mom gave me some Alka-Seltzer a little while ago..."

Mac kept talking, then counting, then was silent for a moment. She dabbed Nancy's forehead again. By now Nancy had stopped her moaning and lay still.

"How many potato chips did you eat?" I asked.

"I guess too many," she answered.

"Feel any better?"

"Yes," her voice sounded exhausted.

Mac looked up at me. "Her pulse is normal now, but I'd keep a check on her. If the pain comes back, no matter what time, we'll get a doctor here. I rather think this is the last case of these pains she will have for a long time." Mac looked Nancy square in the eyes and said, "No more 'pigging out,' kid. I'll check with you tomorrow afternoon."

CHAPTER EIGHT

The Days Begin

Our days began. And it did seem as if every day there was another hurdle to pass. Some were easier than others. Friends continually gave their advice on what to do, what not to do. I knew, as kind as they were to offer, Nancy and I, by trial and error, would have to work together as a team through all the kinks. As much as I wanted one, there was no instruction manual. No one could do this for us. We would be inseparable for at least the next six months.

After a few days Nancy begged me to shampoo her hair. Immediately I regretted not insisting on getting it cut short, but never the less, we had to work out a solution.

"Mom, why don't you scoot me to the side of the bed where my head can be on the edge?" Nancy suggested.

"But I don't want to hurt you," I replied.

"Come on, mom. You're not going to hurt me. And besides, I can almost roll on my side by myself."

Slowly I maneuvered her to the edge, her long hair spilling free. I filled several large pans with warm water and began. As I lathered her hair with shampoo she let out a contented, "Oohh! Mom! This feels so good!"

After several good rinsings I towel dried Nancy's hair, then brushed it out to make sure there were no tangles. Each week Nancy looked forward to her "beauty salon" experience.

By the end of the first week, Fred and I were exhausted. I was not sleeping well, waking every hour or so, still afraid I would not hear Nancy if she called out to us. Each day was filled with working with Nancy to keep her comfortable. Her cast was so heavy I could scarcely lift her to put on her fresh muumuus each morning. We were still trying to settle into some kind of a routine. Nancy, so far, was keeping a good attitude.

Several days later, a box arrived with two beige and

green portable plug-in intercoms. Beautiful! They could have been sky blue and pink and been just as beautiful. We were like three kids trying them out.

"Speak," Fred said from Nancy's room.

"What?" I asked from the other end of the house.

"Anything. The Pledge of Allegiance. Sing the Star Spangled Banner. Anything!"

Instead, I felt like a cheerleader. "Hip, hip, hooray!"

"MOM! It works!" came Nancy's voice. "It's great! This is so neat!"

We left her unit on her bedside table, the second I moved from room to room as I worked, then into our bedroom at night. Now she could order her steaks and cokes via intercom, could keep me posted on the latest news or soap opera story on television and could answer her phone and relay messages if I happened to be outside. When I finished the bedtime routine, just before turning out her light, I pressed the ON button so I would be able to hear any sound from then until morning. I began resting easier at night.

One night soon after, we'd all gone to bed and were asleep. I awoke to the sound of her telephone. In my half sleep I heard Nancy's voice.

"Hello? Hello? Oh, Aunt Bette. Oh, what's wrong?" A moment of silence, then the clink of the receiver. "MOM! DAD! Quick! It's Uncle Dick!

We groped for the light, then made for her room.

"What's wrong?"

"It's Uncle Dick. Aunt Bette wants you to take him to the hospital. He's having a heart attack!"

In moments Fred was dressed and gone. I sat on the edge of Nancy's bed talking until after three. There was little sleep the rest of the night until Fred returned. Dick was having tests and would be kept under observation for a few days, but he did make a full recovery. Somehow our little intercoms had become our best friends.

I felt at times as if I was right back where I was when Nancy was little. I kept saying, "Now, darling, drink your milk. And you must finish your eggs and bacon and juice. If you don't, how will your bones grow strong and straight?"

Now, more than ever, it was important that she eat properly for the fusion to take and bridge over with her own bone to become strong enough to carry her weight for the rest of her life. I remembered the little girl sitting in the high chair, fighting me all the way when I tried to make her finish her oatmeal, or strained beef, or...

I tried to carefully plan each meal. Not only to make it as healthy and delicious as possible, but also easy for Nancy to feed herself. All the while, I tried to keep in mind foods that would not upset her stomach. The night she had become so sick still scared me and I wanted to avoid a repeat. I tried to follow Mac's advice and avoid too many starchy foods or let her chew gum. Both had a tendency to create gas and gas was nearly impossible to get up when lying flat.

Eating while in a prone position was not an easy task, but Nancy quickly learned how to feed herself without spilling too much. We soon found out that smaller meals spaced every couple of hours worked better than three large meals. With the tight fit of the body cast there was not much room for her stomach to expand. I kept her supplied with large plastic glasses of ginger ale and water, buying flexible straws by the carton full.

After several weeks Nancy started complaining of itchy skin. I tried to wash her back as far down in the cast as I could, but it seemed never to be enough. When the itching became unbearable, I knew I had to find a solution. I found a long, thin paintbrush and wrapped it with sterile gauze. I sprinkled baby powder down her cast, then carefully slid the gauze-covered handle in between her cast and her back, gently rubbing the powder into her skin. I avoided the area of her scar, not wanting to risk any type of infection. This seemed to ease the itching. I knew it was not very scientific or medically correct, but it worked. What was the old saying? *"Necessity is the mother of invention."* My only fear was somehow losing the paintbrush down her cast and not being able to retrieve it.

In all honesty, I must admit some days were better than others, some days were worse. On one particular day Nancy was not quite herself. I moved something on her dresser and she shouted, "Leave that alone! It's mine!"

Outbursts were very rare for her and I turned away, not wanting her to see the tears in my eyes or how much she had hurt me.

In an instant she was over her frustration and said, "Oh, mom. I'm so sorry. When this is all over you can go to bed for a month and I will take care of you! Okay?"

"Okay," I answered. In all my lifetime I don't think I could ever have felt a greater depth of love and closeness to my daughter than I did at that moment, but I also couldn't help but smile at the doubtful possibility of that ever happening.

The highlight of each day was Nancy's friends stopping by. School and church friends came often. They laughed and made light of her situation. There were also the times of quiet prayer.

Jill and Pam, along with their boyfriends, came as often as they could. I always kept extra brownies and chocolate chip cookies for Pam's boyfriend, Ken. With both girls preparing for college, their visits became less and less. I could see the envy in Nancy's eyes, knowing she would be confined to home while most of her friends were starting their first year of college; some close by, but most far away.

One evening Stephanie brought her boyfriend, Tommy, and another boy over to visit. I thought everything went fine until the boys were leaving and I overheard Tommy's friend say, "Boy, I sure feel sorry for her."

I hoped Nancy had not heard him, but she had. She angrily lashed out loud enough for him the hear, "Don't ever bring him back! I don't want people to feel sorry for me! I want people to be happy for me!"

Youth can be outspoken when hurt. I felt sorry for both Nancy and the young man. Needless to say, we never saw him again.

The days passed slowly, taking on a sameness. I often thought to myself, *if they seem slow to me, how much slower must they seem to Nancy?* Breakfast, sponge bath, mid morning snack, lunch, mid afternoon snack, Nancy's small television always on, the volume turned low, unless there was a particular program she was interested in. Most evenings Fred and I joined Nancy in her room for dinner. We dined on paper plates, pretending we were on a picnic somewhere.

But each day did pass with the little ups and downs, the many panic buttons that almost got pushed, yet not quite. Each day, as it passed, led us one day closer to the end of the beginning.

It was one of those sticky late August days when the usual trade winds deserted us and the air was close and pressing. I went back and forth between Nancy's room and the kitchen, doing all the usual things that needed doing. I loved the moments when I could sit in her cool of her room with her and watch television, but then I would remember another part of the house that needed attention.

I was back in the kitchen, thinking of starting dinner when I smelled it. Faint at first, then stronger. Smoke! It was close. Not the smell of distant burning brush. More like papers or cloth. Straight down the hall I went, bursting into Nancy's room.

"That you mom?" she said before I entered her view.

"Yes." I quickly looked around but everything seemed okay. I muttered something about forgetting something or other and asked if she needed anything.

"No, mom. Steph will be here in a few minutes."

I left quickly and closed her door tightly. The smell seemed stronger in the hall and in our bedroom. As I began to enter, I heard the familiar call, this time quite urgent.

"Mrs. Webster! Mrs. Webster! Come quick!" Stephanie bolted in the front door trying to muffle her urgency.

I followed her outside and around the side of our house. Under our bedroom window flames leapt up from behind the bushes. A neighbor boy, unaware of our presence, was rumpling papers, throwing them on the flames, his eyes gleeful with mischievousness. A book of matches stuck half way out of his back pocket.

A terror rose up in my heart to meet the anger in my head. I shouted, "In God's name! What are you doing?"

He came out of his trance and jumped back, then forward, stomping the flames. "Oh! Oh!" he stammered. "Oh! Oh! I was just trying to put out this fire!"

By then his mother had heard the commotion and ran out her front door.

"Mama! I didn't start the fire. I was just trying to put it out."

She nodded, "Of course, son. I believe you."

I knew anything I added would be of no use whatsoever. I couldn't fight parental blindness. I couldn't do what I so desperately had the urge to do, whale the tar out of him.

His mother looked over at me and asked, "Did you *see* him start the fire?"

"No, I didn't see him start it."

I wanted to add, *"but I saw him feeding it."* But, it would have accomplished nothing. She chose to believe what she wanted to believe. I knew my only defense and safeguard was vigilance. And I would have to do that as long as Nancy lay completely helpless in her cast in her room at the end of the hall.

Stephanie and I dug the burned papers into the ground and returned to the house.

"Hiya kid!" She bounced into Nancy's room as if nothing had happened, as if the whole world were sunny and good. We had willed it to be so. We wouldn't let Nancy think otherwise.

As each day left us we marked it off Nan's calendar. Three months, twelve weeks, eighty-four days. Eighty-four days sounded better. But all too soon, boredom became our biggest battle. I remembered Dr. Keiser's words, and Mac's as well. Boredom was the one thing we would have to fight. And fight it we did.

But what could an eighteen-year-old possibly accomplish lying flat on her back? We started with books, but holding them up in a position comfortable to read for any length of time was a problem. Television could entertain only for so long. Steph came over every day and tried to keep Nancy's spirits up, but she and I soon began running out of ideas.

One day Nancy asked, "Mom, could you get me some paper, paints, and a new paintbrush?"

My mind buzzed. How could she possibly paint? That evening Fred stayed with Nancy while I drove down to our local Woolworth's. I checked the small arts and crafts section, deciding on a paint by numbers kit. Satisfied with my purchase and feeling just a little guilty of my joy at being out of the house for awhile, I headed home.

Nancy was excited with my choice of canvas imprinted with the outlines of beautiful sleek horses in a summer field, their manes flowing back, caught by the wind, as they cantered across the grass. She laid the canvas against her bent knees, and I set jars of paint on a well worn terry cloth towel beside her. With each brush stroke she gave an extra effort of love. She couldn't ride, nor would she for a very long time, but now she could somehow touch what was in her heart.

Her next project was to plan the redecorating of her room. With pencil and paper she lay on her side scribbling plans and figures.

"When I get out of this I'm going to redecorate completely."

"Redecorate? Good," I said. "Good."

"Now that I'm not riding, with that money and what I have saved, by the time I get out of this, I'll have enough to do everything over."

"Fine," I said. "Get it all figured out. Besides, I could reuse your terry curtains. We're getting low on towels."

Nancy was cool in her little sanctuary. Cool and reasonably comfortable with her air conditioner, her television and princess phone. We continued to communicate via the portable intercoms. It became a game to us.

"Hey, mom! What's for lunch? Hey, mom! Get me my paints please."

Nancy next asked for knitting needles and yarn.

"Knitting needles and yarn?" I asked.

"Sure, mom. I want to knit dad a sweater for Christmas."

I decided not to discourage her. I provided her with what she needed and she began to work. Amazingly it was easy for Nancy to hold the needles up. Click, click, back and forth, row upon row. At times she rested her elbows against her cast. I marveled at her patience, the counting and twisting and marking off, keeping the yarns straight. To her it was a challenge, not for challenge sake, but rather a kind of demon she had to overcome. As if by completing something difficult, she could, in a way, not lose pace with advancing life around her.

That summer of 1965 was hot. Nothing unusual. It was always hot in the summertime. But with the heat came the humidity and tightness of compression, the kind of weather I knew would breed a hurricane sooner or later.

The end of August approached and with it the ski sweater began to take shape. So, also, did a hurricane named Betsy take shape, born off the coast of Trinidad.

CHAPTER NINE

Hurricane Betsy

Sunday evening, September 5, 1965, Fred entered our bedroom where I sat reading in the comfort of air conditioning.

"She's turned clear around! She's coming back!"

"You mean Betsy?" I looked at him in disbelief. "You've got to be kidding!"

He shook his head.

"But hurricanes don't do that!"

"Maybe not. But this one is. She's heading south now, straight for the Bahamas."

Since Betsy's birth as a full-fledged hurricane on August 27, we had been aware of her north and west wavering course. To our initial relief, she passed well east of the Bahamas, still headed north. Then she stalled, three hundred miles east of Cape Kennedy. Usually when a hurricane stalled, it was getting ready to change direction. I had been charting her path on a map cut from the Miami Herald. Not that I was alarmed, but with Nancy in her cast, laying completely immobile in her bed, the thought occurred to me more than once, *what if something happened and we had to get her out fast?*

"What will we do?" I asked.

"We'll get a good night's sleep," Fred answered. "Betsy's a day away. Besides, she's headed for the Bahamas and Cuba, not us. So, relax."

The next morning we awoke to gray skies. The air felt close and damp. Official reports confirmed Betsy's continued path south-southwest.

When I carried Nancy's breakfast tray in to her she was holding her transistor radio to her ear.

"Hi, mom. Guess what?"

"I know," I said, as I set the tray carefully on the side of her bed.

"Maybe we'll get some excitement around here. A hurricane would be a blast!"

I helped her roll onto her side. She bent the straw down and began to drink her orange juice.

"A hurricane IS a blast," I said as I pressed the palm of my hand against her cheek and pushed a wisp of her hair out of the way. Despite her painting and knitting projects, she had become bored with her four pink walls. But a hurricane was a blast we could do without.

Betsy was a massive storm, with an eye over sixty miles across and winds reaching out over three hundred miles in all directions. We were getting gusts already. From Nancy's north and east facing windows I could see that our orange and lime trees had lost some small twigs and leaves. Betsy was poky too, with a forward speed of less than seven miles an hour. No matter where she went, we would feel her breath for some time.

Because of the storm's wide sweep, her 140 mile an hour winds and our close proximity to the Bahamas, at eleven o'clock that Labor Day morning, Miami's hurricane flags were hoisted. Soon hammering sounds could be heard as our neighbors began boarding up. In our neighborhood, when storms approached, people checked on one another. Coffee pots set perking on stoves for a quick cup together before continuing the preparations.

"Will you move Nancy from her room?" One concerned friend asked.

"No. We're going to board up the windows and move her bed to an inside wall."

Hardly had Fred spoken the words when Nancy's windows were covered with sheets of plywood and helping hands moved her bed to a safer spot in her room.

I filled our bathtubs and as many jugs as I could with water. Fred gassed up the car. Just in case. Nancy's wooden makeshift stretcher was stored under her bed, ready if we needed it.

We kept the radio and television on to catch the latest advisories. Ahead of the storm the weather seemed to change dramatically. One moment low dense clouds would unleash heavy rain squalls, the next moment the sky would break away to sunshine. The birds seemed to have vanished.

Were they smarter than we were? There were moments of stillness, quiet and peace. Then came the inevitable rush of wind, dark clouds and torrential rain.

Late that afternoon, Fred and I stood outside nailing the last sheet of plywood in place.

"Mom! Dad!" Nancy called over her intercom. "Betsy's pounding Great Abaco right now!"

Great Abaco, northern most island in the Bahamas, took a beating. By evening it was evident that Betsy was tormenting us. She lumbered toward Nassau, reaching famous Bay Street and Rawson Square at midnight. There she decided to stay awhile, battering the island in another of her temperamental stalls. We were up and down all night, listening to the latest advisories. When she decided to move again we were anxious to know where.

At daybreak on Tuesday, Betsy was still lashing Nassau. Uncertainty hung over us. The winds were wearing down our patience. We were only 145 miles from the center and had been getting strong gusts for hours. When I went into Nancy, she closed her eyes to her boarded windows and made a blind stab at her sheets.

"I wish Betsy'd make up her mind."

"I do too, dear," I answered.

By two o'clock that afternoon Betsy did just that.

Fred and I were sitting in our kitchen having coffee with Maud and Don, Steph keeping Nan company, when the emergency bulletin came in. The storm had begun to move due west toward the Florida coast. Straight for us! Civil Defense advised evacuation of the Keys up to and including Key Biscayne, not many miles from where we lived.

"She's coming! She's coming! Everyone listen!" Nancy's voice blared over the intercom.

"Roger," I acknowledged with attempted flippancy.

"It sounds bad," Don said. "Wish we could keep in touch in case the power and phones go out tonight. If you need me to help move Nancy, or anything, I'd get across the street somehow."

"We can." Fred got up and found his walkie-talkies. He handed one to Don.

From two o'clock on the winds steadily increased.

The sky turned an eerie yellow-gray. To the east, over the Gulf Stream, Betsy was heading toward us. Once she picked up speed there would be no stopping her. By late afternoon we could no longer venture outside. Each home on our block was boarded up, cars parked on the leeward side of each. The street was eerily deserted.

The air hung heavy and we used the hall fan to try and circulate some fresh air. Fred and I dined on the edge of Nancy's bed, trying to laugh and make light of Betsy's unwanted visit. Darkness came earlier than usual. By seven o'clock the only thing we could see from our front door were sheets of rain, and just beyond, the branches of our ficus tree pointed to the west as Betsy's winds whipped through them.

I made use of every minute, getting my days work done and Nancy settled comfortably for the night. *There's just no telling, no telling at all.* The same thought crept in every time, once you've lived through a hurricane. I tried to still the thought as I slipped a fresh muumuu over Nancy's outstretched arms and down over her cast.

"Anything special you want?" I finished brushing her hair.

"Mmm. Some brownies, coke and my transistor radio. Please."

"As you wish."

My, weren't we the essence of politeness.

I turned to check the glass jalousie windows. The plywood on the outside helped secure them against the rising gusts. I returned to the kitchen to fill Nancy's snack tray.

At ten-thirty the first hurricane winds hit and from then on there was no let up. From 75 miles per hour, to 100, to 125. The winds slammed twigs, leaves, bits of rock and sand against the house. Each successive gust seemed to jar the very foundation and tore at the roof. A gravel sound hit the east windows, then a rush of wind followed by thumps. At eleven the center of Betsy was still over seventy miles away and even though she had picked up speed, it would be hours before the eye passed over us. It felt like we were huddling in a pothole of earth, waiting for hell to pass over.

At midnight Don checked in with us on the walkie-talkie Fred had given him.

"How's it going over there?"

"Okay, so far. The metal shutters on our patio door are beating pretty badly. Sure hope the screws hold. How about you?"

"Water's coming in under the utility room door, but Maud and Stephanie are keeping ahead of it. How's our gal taking all this?"

"Like a trooper," Fred answered.

From then on we called back and forth frequently. We kept up our vigil, going from room to room, checking windows and doors. As the gusts whipped at the patio door storm shutters, they bent in and out, making a strange tinny sound. The bottom screws had loosened and we prayed the rest would hold. Sheet metal could be razor sharp in flight.

There was no sense in trying to sleep. We could only wait it out. We listened as the wind roared down the power lines out back, tore through the trees and shrubs, grinding melaleuka branches against the corner of the roof. Time seemed to inch by.

Shortly after three in the morning Nancy called out to us. "Betsy's coming in at Key Largo! She's almost here! Please come in here with me?"

We rushed in. Fred sat in the wing back chair. I half reclined on Nancy's bed. With Betsy's latest slight turn we would remain just outside and due north of the hurricane eye and would not see a center calm, only winds like nothing we could ever have imagined. Time seemed to stand still as Betsy rushed at our home with a deafening roar.

I leaned over to straighten the sheet atop Nancy's cast. Fred sensed my uneasiness.

"The roof won't go," he said. "These cement block houses can take two hundred mile an hour winds. Miami's building code. Remember?"

"That's good, Dad," Nancy said with a half smile, then flicked up the volume on the radio.

We listened to the reports as they came in. The Keys and South Miami were getting the brunt of the storm. Power out. Severe flooding. Many trees down. Beach front hotels with sand and water in their lobbies. Sea walls crumbling like children's blocks.

Our lights flickered off, then on, then finally off. I lit my granny's old oil lamp and Fred kept his flashlight by his side. To pass the time we tried to guess what was hitting the plywood covering Nancy's east window. A branch? Leaves? Sand? Scraping, thumping, grating. Would our house ever be quiet again?

Minutes slowly slipped away into hours. At last, gray flecks of dawn filtered through the cracks around Nancy's windows. It was well after six a.m. when, for one split second, the wind seemed to stop. The worst was over. Exhaustion had caught up with Nancy. I gently slipped the transistor radio from her sleep relaxed fingers and we left her to slumber.

Our home had weathered another hurricane. From its tight, dry safeness we looked out at a world gray and beaten.

It was not until five p.m. that afternoon that the hurricane flags finally came down, fifty-four long hours after they had first been hoisted.

CHAPTER TEN

After the Hurricane

We were lucky. Our only major damage from Betsy was two downed melaleuka trees that had fallen across our chain link fence, leaving a big dent. One tree still stood, but had rubbed the metal gutter into a down-spout. That must have been the scraping sound we heard from Nancy's room. Other than that we had a few big branches down and leaves stuck like glue to the sides of the house.

After breakfast I went outside and began hosing the leaves off the walls. Fred came out and took the hose from my hand.

"You have enough to do with Nancy. I'll take care of it." He began removing the boards covering the windows, letting the sunshine in once more.

When I went in to check on Nancy, she excitedly said, "Mom! I can still see one of my trees. At least they're not all gone." I smiled at the thought that such a simple thing could make her so happy.

For Nancy's sake, as well as our own, we tried to return to normal as quickly as possible.

Steph started her senior year of high school. Even so, she came over each morning before school to have breakfast with Nan, always entering the bedroom with a big smile and her "Hiya kid" greeting. Steph returned most afternoons with her homework, Nan helping her as much as she could. She was a lifesaver to me, staying with Nancy in the afternoons so that I could get out a bit to the store or bank. I didn't want to leave Nancy for too long, but I knew with Steph she was in good hands.

At least once a week Steph came to me and asked the inevitable question, "Are you going to bake another apple pie, Mrs. Webster?"

That was the only thing she ever asked me for and I gladly complied, always keeping extra apples in the fridge.

She loved to stand in the kitchen and watch me peel the apples, then roll out the dough. Mama had taught me how to peel an apple without breaking the peel, and Steph asked more than once, "How do you do that, Mrs. Webster?" I'd smile as I piled the apples high into the bottom portion of dough, adding cinnamon and butter before topping it with the remaining dough.

Steph would return from Nancy's room when I pulled the pie from the oven, taking two hot slices back to share with Nan, always adding her, "Thanks, Mrs. Webster!"

Weekends Steph spent hours at our house. She kept Nancy up to date on what all the kids were doing, what was in and what was not. She was an integral part of our family and we loved her dearly for her patience, love and caring. With Jill and Pam off to college it seemed it all fell on Steph's shoulders, but she never once complained. She always had a smile on her face and tried to keep a smile on Nan's face as well.

Nancy completed another sweater and two more paintings. Several times a week she would ask for her bags of shells. Rolling herself onto her side, she sorted and resorted her shell treasures. She always saved the Angel Wings for last. I would remove them from the black shell box and she would spend several minutes holding them in her hands.

We talked about Sanibel, planning for the next time we'd head over the "Tamiami Trail." How we'd walk the beach again and hunt for more shells and eat and sleep until we were slept out. We'd stand together again, looking out over the water, letting the foam wash over our toes, talking in that changing way, more like two adults. Nancy would come a long way in the next year. A long way in learning patience and understanding and dreaming. But with dreaming came the knowledge that dreams do not always come true.

Even with all her projects and talking of Sanibel, Nancy started to get depressed. There were moments when she admitted she didn't care about anything. I tried to tell her this would pass and soon she would be in her walking cast. I knew we had to do something more for her, but what?

One Sunday Fred and Don helped Nancy roll onto her stretcher, then carried her into the living room, carefully laying her down on an extra mattress I had set on the floor. She was in her glory that day, removed from the four pink walls of her room and with her prism glasses she could watch television with Steph. Dick, Bette and Marilyn came over, staying most of the afternoon and Dick helped carry her back into her bedroom that evening. Nancy commented that if only she could look forward to that on Sundays, she wouldn't mind nearly as much. We repeated the process for the next several Sundays.

We filled the days as best we could and September soon became October. We neared the three-month point in Nancy's recovery and she was scheduled to return to the hospital to have her body cast removed and her walking cast put on. We had been told that the walking cast was a lighter weight cast, which would enable her to walk again and sit for a limited amount of time each day, but it was just as restrictive as the body cast. The fusion of her spine was not yet complete and would not be for another nine months.

Nancy counted down the days, filled with anticipation that she soon would be able to walk again. October 10, the red circled day on the calendar, finally arrived. We reversed the process, gently rolling Nancy back onto her stretcher. As we opened the front door and carried her out to the car, she looked up at the sky.

"Oh! How wonderful! Look at the sky!"

Her joy made me wonder if we should not live our lives just this way, as if what we have and are at the moment never existed before, nor would ever exist again.

We carefully slid her into the back of the station wagon, cushioning her among blankets and pillows. She sang all the way back to the hospital, a little off key, but what did it matter? Her excitement was contagious and I joined in, my voice not much better than hers, but we made our best stab at a duet.

At Variety Children's we checked Nancy in for her three day stay. Returning home we once more faced her empty room, her big double bed devoid of life. The relief from work was not in me at all. I missed her call, "Mom, I'd like a coke!" Or, "Mom, come move me up and over."

Love made work a satisfying accomplishment. To be rid of it was not a feeling of relief, but instead a bit of sadness. For only through loving and doing, that feeling of being needed, could full satisfaction come. I knew this for sure and the room was suddenly too quiet and lonely. I turned off the light, went out and closed the door.

The next day her new cast was to be put on. I asked and was given permission to come downstairs with her. One of the nurses told me she would let me in with Nancy for a few minutes after the new cast was in place. I stood in the hallway outside the cast room where Nancy was, listening to the nearly deafening sound of the cast cutter saw. I could only imagine what it must be like for her, laying there, feeling the vibration of the saw as the doctor cut through the layers of plaster.

I paced the hall waiting for one of the nurses to come and get me. When I finally walked into the cast room, Nancy was still laying on the Stryker frame. I immediately understood why she had been so frightened of falling through the thin strips.

As soon as the plaster was dry, a nurse stood on either side of Nancy and they slowly pulled her up into a sitting position. One of the nurses asked me to stand next to Nan and hold her arm. The nurse kept reminding her to take deep breaths so that she would not pass out. After three months of lying absolutely flat, the abrupt uprighting made her stomach feel queasy and the room moved crazily. Slowly her breathing steadied.

When they were sure she would not faint, one of the nurses took my place. They firmly grasped both her arms and brought her up into a standing position. She trembled as blood rushed to her feet. Again they gave her time to adjust to being upright before encouraging her to take a step.

I held my breath as they assisted her in taking her first steps in over three months. With many helping hands she walked straight and tall down the hospital corridor. I followed close behind. The hospital staff flanked her on both sides, clapping with approval at her shaky but determined steps.

We were told it would take days for her to have the strength and balance to walk on her own. Nancy was learning to walk all over again and I wanted to shout out loud, *"She did it!"* as I had done so many years before.

When everything was to Dr. Keiser's satisfaction, Nancy was returned to her room, where she would spend another night. I sat next to her bed for a while longer. For some reason I felt a sense of letdown, that sinking, helpless feeling. This cast was no different from the first cast. The full realization of that made the truth come through to me. She was going to be almost as confined for the next 84 days as she had been for the past 84 days. Except, that she would be able to walk into another room, see other walls, but she wouldn't be able to walk for long with such a heavy cast on her.

If the realization had come through to her, she did not show it. Her way of holding things in, like her dad, was good in a way, yet perhaps not so. I had no way of knowing. But then as always, her moments of confidence came in spurts and I knew enough to wait for them to come naturally. I knew she would be all right. She had already proven that to me in the last three months. There had been very few moments of feeling sorry for herself, very few complaints about the operation leaving her so immobile.

Mabel took over in helping Nancy practice her walking. Every hour or so she would come into Nancy's room and help her up, take her arm and walk her down the hallway. Later that evening when we called to talk to Nancy, she commented, "Mabel made me get up and walk five times!" Thank goodness she was laughing as she said it.

When I arrived at the hospital the next day, two young boys whizzed into Nancy's room and in between her bed and her roommate's. They seemed like polite, friendly boys. When I later learned they were from Kendall Youth Hall, supposedly delinquents, I could not accept it. Nancy told me the previous night they had come into her room with cokes and goodies, asked if she was all right and could they do anything for her. There was nothing to indicate any sort of bad behavior.

This time, as we left Variety Children's, Nancy sat in

the front seat with me. On the way home she remarked at everything she saw, as if she were seeing things for the first time. I felt as if I was seeing the world in a fresh, new perspective.

"You have no idea how great this is!" Nancy said the next morning as she sat at the kitchen table eating her breakfast.

"Mom."

"Hmm?"

"You know those two boys? They were trying so hard to be good and they were so kind. They need someone to reach them now, before it's too late. Because they really are good kids, but they're on the brink. I wish I could help them."

"Well, perhaps someday you can. Not them in particular, but boys and girls like them. Perhaps social work is what you'd like to head for. There is a place for you wherever you want to be, a need for whatever you want to do. And by their doing for you, we saw their need manifested in doing good acts. If they cannot succeed in this way, then they will turn toward what they have already begun, the downward road. Every human being needs recognition. They got that from you because you appreciated their kindness and they were satisfied for awhile."

"Whew. That's a lot to think about, mom."

Each morning Nancy laughed as I cautioned her, "Please don't get up unless I'm here. You might get woozy and I don't want to pick up hunks of cracked plaster."

Each day Nancy tried walking a little further. First, she walked around the house hanging onto my arm until she felt steady on her feet. Then she ventured out into the backyard. Nancy was diligent about keeping to her twenty minutes a day sitting time. She usually saved her time for dinner when the three of us gathered around the kitchen table. She and I stored our day's stories just for that time when we were all together. Fred, with his big grin, listened intently to our ramblings.

Two weeks later Dr. Keiser called to check on Nancy. "How's my girl?"

"Fine, Dr. Keiser. I'm walking much better now."

"That's good. Keep it up."

One morning Nancy asked, "Mom, could we go the shopping center? Just for a little while? Just to look around?"

163rd Street Shopping Center was not far from our home, but as it was we fudged a little on the twenty-minute a day sitting restriction. I limited the shopping to Burdine's, hoping she would not become too tired. Nancy wanted to look at all the new fashions, but not being able to try anything on, she had to settle for holding skirts and blouses up to her cast. It soon became apparent that other shoppers were staring at her. Whether it was the cast or her bright pink muumuu I am not sure, but she became uncomfortable with the attention. We soon left and did not return to shop until after she was out of her walking cast.

Nancy began her breaking away process in earnest. Although I was still there to assist with bathing and washing hair, there were many things she was now able to do for herself. It felt strange after three months of taking care of every need, every request, but I knew this was how it should be. I let the strings out further and further, but still worried she was trying to do too much. She still tired easily and that kept things to a slower pace. At least for awhile.

Over dinner one night in late October, Nancy made her announcement. "Know what I want to do tonight?"

"No..." her dad and I said at the same time.

"I want to walk over to Steph's."

"Tonight?"

"Sure."

"Do you feel you can go that far?" I asked.

"Sure," she said as she pierced her cucumber salad with her fork.

"Okay. Okay. But not alone," I replied.

"No..." she trailed off in her way that usually denoted a, *but I could if I tried*, undercurrent.

The pitch of her voice, the up or down, had a way of telling me more than the ordinary yes or no. Good. She was becoming independent. We were realizing we would soon have to let go. Not just over to Steph's, but, when this was all over and done with, off to college, possibly a teaching job, marriage. Yes, the pulling away could be seen right down to the tip of her fingers that continued to jab the cucumber unmercifully. And my wanting to hold on, like the way I held on to my coffee cup. I set my cup down and let go, as I knew I would have to in this other way soon. Too soon.

We watched her cross the street that night. Steph met her half way, just in case. From then on it was so good to hear her say again, "Mom! I'm going over to Steph's! Be back later!"

Nancy was scheduled for her six-week check up with Dr. Keiser at his office in Coral Gables. She was self conscious about the trip, not sure what to wear. The night before her appointment, I worked on a corduroy muumuu with long sleeves. My buttonhole attachment chose, at that very moment, to snap a screw. My good neighbor, Dorothy, hauled out her machine and worked up the twelve buttonholes that would have taken me hours to do by hand.

The results of her examination and x-ray? Dr. Keiser's face showed them clearly. He came into the examining room with the biggest grin I've ever seen on a comedian, let alone a stern, efficient, exacting doctor. She hadn't slipped! The past weeks, since she started walking and sitting again, were critical ones. Orders had to be followed right down the line. And Nancy had. Many times she had eaten lunch lying down because she was saving her sitting time for something else.

I felt the weight lift from my shoulders. Although I realized this was not the end of the critical period, it was a very good indication of how things were going to go. When we arrived back home, Nancy went directly to the living room and placed her hands upon the shell box. Then she moved her fingers down until they rested directly over the two Angel Wing shells.

"My Angel Wings," she said.

"Yes," I answered.

Our Angel Wings. Bless them.

I found myself with more time to sit at my typewriter. I had written Dr. Harrington about Nancy. He sent back a kind letter with his good wishes for Nancy's recovery and included the latest information on scoliosis. Surrounding myself with his letter and information I had been gathering, I began, in earnest, my reflections into the past and my attempt to find answers. My fingers began to type as fast as they could, transferring my thoughts into printed words.

CHAPTER ELEVEN

From the Beginning

We can never go back to any part of our lives, except in memory. From the day we faced Nancy's need for surgery, I tried to sift through the high and low points of our lives in an attempt to answer my questions.

How, when and why did this all start?

When I was fifteen, I thought I had life all figured out. Love, marriage and two children. That's what I would have someday. A loving husband and two beautiful, bright, perfect children. A little boy in patched blue jeans and pigtailed little girl in organdy and lace.

Ten years later I married Fred. He came from a typical New England family, conservative in their outlook. That didn't bother me as I had also been raised with a firm hand. His English and Scotch background complemented by conglomeration of nationalities - Swedish, Danish, Irish and the Narragansett Indian my father had always insisted was on his side. I never let on I thought he was only boasting. Later, I found out he was not. His grandmother, my great-grandmother Lydia, was, indeed, half Narragansett Indian. What really mattered was that Fred and I both came from healthy stock. Any offspring of ours would have that in their favor.

From the first moment I saw Fred I knew there could be no one else but this tall, straw haired, quiet mannered fellow. One afternoon during the summer of '42, while visiting my best friend Hilda at her home, I happened to peak out the window and noticed two young fellows walking by. One was tall and handsome, the other shorter and wearing glasses. Both were laughing.

"Who are they?" I asked my friend.

Hilda stood beside me and peaked out. "The tall one is Freddy. The other one is his friend, Donald." She jokingly added, "Which one do you choose?"

"Freddy." It seemed to me I didn't even have to think about it.

Hilda opened her front door and called out, "Freddy! Donald! I want you to meet my friend Arlene!"

Freddy and Donald stopped, turned around and walked back up Hilda's driveway. The four of us sat down on the wide cement steps.

Hilda made the proper introductions.

"Freddy, Donald, this is Arlene. She works at Dr. Fish's."

In a quiet voice, Freddy said, "Hi Arlene."

Donald, who I would come to know as the comic, piped up, "Hey, Arlene! What about me?"

I turned, smiled at him and said, "Hi Donald."

"Whose car is that?" Freddy looked over at my Model A roadster with the rumble seat. "Nice car."

"My brother fixed it up and gave it to me. I've named her Betsy."

Freddy smiled a big smile.

Donald sat back with a smile on his face. He knew. And I knew even then who my heart belonged to.

College and World War II came between us for the next several years. I did not hear from Fred again until I received a letter from him during December '44. Home from college on my Christmas break, we had had one of our typical winter snowstorms. A time to stay indoors and keep warm, but mama wanted her mail.

I told her I would go for her and she said, "Put on your snow boots, mittens and warm hat, dear girl."

I did and shuffled my way up the long driveway, past pure white snow drifts almost as high as the top of papa's garage door. When I opened the box and pulled out the cold, soggy mail I saw a letter addressed to Arlene Miller from Frederick Clark Webster. My heart kept skipping beats as I sloshed back to the house and stomped the snow from my boots. Mama was just putting an apple pie into the oven of her black wood stove and the kitchen was toasty warm. I sat down and ripped open the envelope.

Dear Arlene,

Still in the service, but would like to see you when I come home next month on leave.

Fred

During a long weekend in January of '45 the whole gang got together again. Donald, Hilda, Hilda's sister Ella, Freddy and me. Then Fred was off again. Back to the war.

VJ Day. August 15, 1945. Will any of us ever forget? Hilda, Ella and I were in Boston and were soon caught up in all the celebrating; crowds of people like I had never seen before. But the only thing on my mind was, *when would I see Fred again?*

That fall I received another short letter from Fred. He would be home on furlough and wanted to get together. We spent several glorious days driving through Vermont, talking about our hopes and dreams, getting to know one another. And we did keep it all very proper, staying in separate cabins.

It was another six months before Fred was home for good. The girls told me he had gotten home on April 26. I waited, but he didn't call.

I was crushed.

In mid May we met by chance and climbed up Chickatawbut Tower with another couple. We talked and talked, catching up with one another's happenings. However, the evening ended with no future date.

Early June, Ella and I went to the theater. Halfway through the movie, Freddy and Donald came up the balcony steps. They'd seen my roadster parked outside and had come looking for us. My heart did flip-flops as we four walked out of the theater. After stopping for sandwiches at Boots and Saddles, we rode around until after midnight.

A week later, Ella and I were visiting Hilda. The fellows stopped by. We four took off for Nantasket Beach to ride the roller coaster and Ferris wheel. We walked the beach, then stopped for ice cream at Howard Johnson's. There still was no future date planned.

At the end of June, with a week of vacation time, I boarded a train for Colorado Springs to visit my dear friend Doris Jean.

Early July, Ella and I bumped into the boys down

near Blue Hills. Freddy and I ended up going canoeing. We stopped at the Shady Nook for sandwiches and soda. Afterward we drove for miles in my roadster. When we pulled up in front of his house, Freddy said, "How about Wednesday night?" I gave him my *it's okay* smile.

On our first "official date" we took in a movie. Our goodnight included plans for the beach the next Saturday.

We enjoyed our beach date, then saw each other nearly every day for the next week and a half. We visited friends, went dancing, drove to New Hampshire, went to the movies, and drove to visit friends in Montague.

The happiest day of my life was the day Fred asked me to marry him. July 22, 1946, we were kissing goodnight after a date. Fred smiled at me and said, "Let's do what Russ and my sister Marion just did."

My breath caught on my words, "You're asking me to marry you?"

"Yes," he answered. "But not to drive up to New Hampshire to do it. Let's make it a church wedding with all the trimmings."

I remembered back to the time I had asked my mother how I would know when I was in love. Mama's words were simply, "My dear girl, you will know when you no longer have to ask."

My head was spinning. My heart went lub-a-dub. My answer was a direct and sure, "Yes." There were no doubts.

We talked and talked, deciding on an autumn wedding. That night as I drove the six miles home, I kept repeating aloud, "Mrs. Frederick Clark Webster. I'll be Mrs. Frederick Clark Webster."

Several days later, Fred took me home to his mother and said, "Mom, Arlene and I are planning to get married."

She put her arms around me, smiled and said, "Welcome to our family."

She not only opened her arms to me, but her home as well. From that day on I felt special, like a chosen child. Never once did she seem like a mother-in-law, never once did she criticize. She always treated me with fairness and love.

I was in a near panic during the hectic months before we were married. There were the invitations to send out, the white satin gown with white satin bows and white satin slippers to check and recheck, choosing the flowers and decorations for the church and convincing the minister that white bows and candles down the aisle pews would be quite safe.

Despite all the preparations, we managed to spend several weekends in Vermont looking for a farm to buy. Fred's and my dream was to own land and a big farmhouse to raise our family. Unfortunately, we never did find just the right property.

On October 5, 1946, in a traditional 7 p.m. candlelight ceremony in a picturesque, white New England church, Fred and I said our vows. Fred's brother, Dick, was his best man and Hilda was my matron of honor. Candles flickered on the altar inside, while outside a harvest moon shown down from a clear autumn sky.

If my heart had not been as sturdy as it was, I am sure it would have burst with the happiness I felt walking down the red carpeted aisle in the very church where I had been baptized and attended Sunday School. I was now about to take the most serious of vows before God. I kept repeating to myself, *This is it! This is it! This is what I had been waiting for all my life!* If I could only hold this very moment forever. I pressed my fingers against my palm, as if to grasp the fleeting seconds. But I knew I couldn't when I saw Fred standing at the altar. Suddenly I wanted to hurry on toward him.

Only one blunder marred the perfection of the ceremony. Fred, in his excitement, forgot to kiss me at the altar. The organist waited. The pastor waited. All our guests waited. Fred grinned at me, so I stood waiting too. He turned, took my arm in the crook of his elbow and we headed down the center aisle.

We were halfway down the stairs to the reception when he called after me, "Hey, Arlene! Wait a minute! I forgot something!" He took me in his arms, gave me a big kiss and said, "Hello, Mrs. Webster!"

And that is who I became and knew I would be forever. Each of our guests coming down the stairs behind us clapped, adding their congratulations. We enjoyed our church reception with our three-tiered wedding cake and ice-cream. Punch was served from a cut glass bowl with a silver ladle, an old family heirloom.

We returned to my mother's house to change. While Hilda helped me into my going away clothes, a blue suit I had made on mama's old treadle sewing machine, the "boys" were outside tying tin cans onto the back bumper of our car along with a Just Married sign.

As Fred and I pulled away, mama, with tears in her eyes, waved and called after us, "Be happy! And be good to each other!"

We waved back and said we would. And we were for the rest of our life together.

We left on a five-day honeymoon touring New England and Canada, including Niagara Falls. As his wedding gift, my brother, Sonny, put a new motor in my '31 roadster and mama bought four new tires.

With gas at eleven cents a gallon, Fred and I covered many miles enjoying beautiful Indian summer weather. The countryside was a mass of vivid and blending colors. The maples, birches, elms and oaks splashed shades of red, orange, yellow, green and brown across the whole horizon. The air was sweet and warm by day and at night there was the crisp and pungent smell of the earth in fields recently turned over waiting for the coming winter and spring beyond.

If spring brought hope and promise of new life, then fall and our beginning brought a happiness and hope not dependent upon any set time. We were two people beginning a new life together and were like no other two people in the world. Sunrises and sunsets existed solely for us. The iciness of the clear mountain streams, the quiet back lanes, the friendliness of little towns was for our pleasure exclusively. We stopped at wayside gift shops and bought fresh picked Macintosh apples for munching along the way. We indulged in hot fudge sundaes at an old drug store where counter stools squeaked when we spun around in them.

We talked and dreamed and planned.

At Niagara Falls, we boarded the Maid of the Mist. Our gear was oil slickers and Nor'Easters. From the deck we stood entranced at the magnificence of the falls. That day, unlike all the others, was gray with a low cloud mass. Mist dampened my face and sent a chill through me. Then, suddenly, looking at each other, the chill went away.

Premonition? Who could ever determine the significance of what we feel at any given moment? If no more than the sign that all of life could not be blue skies and cloudless days, that was it. That somewhere along the way we would know a chill, a gray day or two, but together, we could make it go away.

Returning home, we spent our first night at mom and pop's. Over breakfast the next morning, mama had a big surprise for us. She told us that the Cape Cod house around the corner on Coney Street was vacant and we could stay there as long as we needed to. The house was a cozy two bedroom, with a fireplace and large screened in porch. With some extra furniture mama had, Fred and I moved into our first home together. Both of us continued to work.

Two children did I say? I was a bit off in my planning. When our first and only child decided on coming to us, I knew the baby's intention long before medical science could have proved me right or wrong. Mothers-to-be have a way of knowing.

One evening, a few months later at a Grange supper, my dear friend Hilda leaned over the table and whispered, "You're going to have a baby, aren't you?"

"Yes. But how on earth did you know?"

Hilda smiled, "I could tell by your eyes and your face. There's a glow."

She was right. There was a glow from happiness like no other. A few months later when I felt that tiny being begin to move, I knew God had placed His hand upon my shoulder, charging me with a responsibility unlike any I'd had before. Accepting my responsibility, I followed the doctor's advice right down the line. Plenty of rest, exercise and good food, and I took no medications of any kind.

From the beginning I felt like shouting the news from every street corner and in every store. One day I entered a fabric shop. "Do you have cotton batiste and flannelette? I'm going to have a baby and I must get started making things." The sales clerk smiled as she reached for the bolts of fabric.

In the days ahead I made a layette right down to the flannelette diapers, cut with extra sharp pinking shears. When completed, I carefully folded each article and placed it in the second hand maple chest Fred had bought and refinished. Often I spent time in the tiny upstairs bedroom that was to become the nursery, taking out every piece of clothing, refolding it and then putting it back again. I stood by the crib and ran my fingers over the top rail, thinking, dreaming. Will my child ever be big enough to outgrow this bed? Will he stand tall and straight?

Like any prospective parent, I prayed our child would be physically and mentally perfect. Beautiful features were secondary to the beauty I hoped he would develop within. Just let our child have two sturdy legs and a straight back to stand up to this world and its demands. Two strong hands to work, play and comfort others. Two eyes to catch the glistening of a raindrop on a blade of grass. Two ears to hear the needs of man and the music he can make. A mind to take in, weigh, sift, then give out clearly and honestly. Two lips I hoped would seldom cause pain. And a heart, big, wide and open.

Aware of my own shortcomings, I knew my child would also not be perfect.

During those months of anticipation, only one question popped into my head without being answered. Would my job, in any way, cause harm to my baby? As assistant to a chemist in a textile plant, I worked with vinyl and cellulose, perfecting formulae for waterproofing fabrics. The lab was light and airy. The work was pleasant. I stayed until my eight month. Often, since, I have wondered if this had any bearing in later years.

CHAPTER TWELVE

The Early Years

Saturday, July 19 came early for me. About four in the morning I awoke with a twitching pain. Excitement rose in my throat. Perhaps today our child would be born. The pain went away, I laid back and fell asleep. When I awoke with another twitch, I knew my excitement would not let me drift off again. An hour or more passed, my oneness with the silence slowly dissipating as black turned to gray, then dawn; the sun's rays beginning to filter through our organdy curtained windows. The room was cool, but I knew it would not be for long.

Downstairs in our kitchen, our old icebox dripped water faster than ever into the pan below. *If only our shiny new refrigerator would come today.* In 1947 we were still in the midst of the aftermath of the war, still feeling the effects of shortages of materials and household items. Weeks before when we had ordered the refrigerator Fred had asked the salesman, "Shouldn't we have some kind of priority, seeing as we are expecting a baby?" The salesman promised to do the best he could.

This was to be my day. I sensed it as I stood in the kitchen buttering toast. The twitching pains were coming about an hour apart. In between, I almost forgot. No need to bother anyone yet. Besides, there was much to be done. Ironing, baking, tying up loose ends that would be untied soon enough.

Hour after hour I busied myself. At three that afternoon, I began to wonder why my child was so persistently persistent in keeping our status as it had been all day. Would he be a balky, stubborn child? One we would have to prod and scold? Perhaps, instead, he would be the quiet contemplative type that didn't want to rush anything, including being born.

Shortly after, the appliance store truck pulled into

our drive. I momentarily forgot my musings. Such a beauty was that white giant the men wheeled into our kitchen. Out the door went the old dripping icebox with a helpful push from me. The new refrigerator hummed softly when we plugged it in. Opening the large white door, I peered in to the space where I could place my already melting butter and sagging Jell-O. Plenty of room for baby formula, extra milk, and all the foods our baby would need to grow tall and strong.

Somehow my time seemed to stand still. Twelve hours now since the first twitching pain and still no change. In a burst of energy I made a batch of homemade frozen ice-cream custard. With egg beaters whirling and the counter top thoroughly messed up, our kitchen looked like that of a hostess frantically preparing for a grand party.

After supper, Fred and I tried to relax on our screened porch, he up and down from the glider, me filling the lawn chair. Even the creamy frozen custard we enjoyed only distracted our thoughts for a little while.

"Something must be wrong," Fred said. "I'm going to call the doctor. I think we should get you to the hospital and find out."

"Nothing's wrong," I quipped. "Nature's first try is usually a bit slow, that's all." I turned away, inwardly not so sure of my words.

Sunday, July 20, at three in the morning, after almost twenty-four hours of initial labor, our child finished clowning around and was getting ready to enter our world.

"Come on," Fred said nervously.

I took a last look around the house. Spying the remains of a bushel of peaches, I grabbed several.

"What are you doing?" he asked.

"Oh, just getting a few to eat on the way," I answered.

He gulped in disbelief, placed my suitcase in the rumble seat of our Model A roadster and helped me climb into the front seat.

"It's such a beautiful night, let's put the top down and ride out to Nantasket Beach," I said. "We could watch the sun come up. Bet we have time!"

Fred ignored my flippancy and turned the key in the

ignition. I leaned my head back to catch the moon full on my face and let the cool breeze brush my hair. What a beautiful night to be born, I thought. What a beautiful night to be born.

Our child had other ideas. He was a she and chose to arrive by day. At one o'clock Sunday afternoon, thirty-three hours after her first hint, Nancy came into our lives.

Fred, in his eagerness to share the news of his new baby girl, sped over the back roads to his mom's house and to his dismay was pulled over. As the policeman started to write out the ticket, Fred excitedly told him about his new daughter. The officer took a moment to verify with the hospital, then tore up the ticket. Looking sternly at Fred, he said, "Young man, I am letting you go. But remember you are a father now. Drive safely and stay alive!"

Fred drove the rest of the way to his mom's several miles under the speed limit and never forgot the officer's words.

How do I describe the first moments with my first child? I peeked at the tiny bundle the nurse placed in my arms. Still very unsure of myself, I held her stiffly, as if she might fall apart.

"May I touch her?"

The nurse smiled, "She's yours, isn't she? Don't worry. Babies are glued together quite well."

I placed my finger on her cheek. My daughter's face felt like soft velvet, soft and fragile. Encircling her with both arms, I held her tight, wondering if anyone else in the world ever felt quite this way. Suddenly the practical, un-dreaming part of me emerged.

"Is she all right?"

"She's fine. And all the parts are working!" The nurse noticed my concern over the forceps mark on Nancy's cheek and nose and the definite point to the back of her head. "Nothing to worry about. It was a long labor. Her head will shape round as she grows and the marks will disappear."

"Pinhead," the nurses all lovingly called her. They gave her extra hugs whenever they placed her in my arms. Each time I held her I would recheck. Ten tiny fingers on well shaped hands. Ten tiny toes at the end of well formed legs. Except for the shape of her head, she looked perfect.

Besides, the doctor would have told us if something were wrong, wouldn't he?

Nine days later Fred drove us home. It didn't take long to realize all was not sweet smooth joy. There were bottles, feedings, diapers, bathing, wondering, worrying. All the unsureness that accompanied any new job of importance.

What do we remember of our children's first weeks and months? Their first cry? First word? First step? I didn't keep a detailed record of Nancy's every response or action. I figured I'd not forget the best, nor the worst of happenings. I was sure my memory would mark them in my mind.

Looking back I remember a cuddly, soft, completely dependent baby. Kicking, always kicking. Little hands continually in motion. I remember a wobbly head and little wisps of light brown hair, a hint of blue in her eyes and a full, round face. She was not dimply, though, but long and slim. Nancy didn't have folds of baby fat, nor did she ever acquire them. She would be tall and thin like her dad and paternal grandmother. She seldom cried and smiled often. She was a happy baby.

What does always come back to me is the difficulty in getting Nancy to eat. She was more content to sleep. A few ounces of milk, a spoonful or two of cereal and she closed her eyes, her head resting securely in the crook of my arm.

Whenever I discussed this with our family doctor, he said, "She's fine."

About that time, Dr. Spock's new theory of permissiveness was just coming into vogue. I couldn't buy the idea entirely. Along with loving discipline, I believed a schedule was necessary for feeding. As in living one's life, there need to be guidelines. Maybe not as strict as the "old school," but a moderate approach at least.

Even so, babies needed love served with their milk. A hug and soft words to help down the cereal and fruit. An old fashioned rocking chair was the best place to offer the duel sustenance. We were lucky. One of our wedding gifts was a Salem rocker. Low, wide, and with a high back, it proved to be a good place for feeding, hugging and soft words. And it did help. Nancy ate a little more, but still not enough to suit me.

"She's healthy. Give her the vitamins and stop worrying." Our doctor was emphatic.

I tried. I would rock, talk and sing. I would say softly, "Please eat. You can't grow straight and strong without eating."

Two months passed, then three. Nancy began to follow sounds and objects. She knew my voice and her father's. She knew the security of our arms.

One afternoon she lay in her carriage on our screened porch. "Come quick!" Fred called to me as I worked in the kitchen. I dropped my dishtowel and ran, sure something had happened.

It had.

Nancy was grinning up at us. In her hand she held a blue heart shaped rattle, waving it back and forth. We didn't know whether or not she realized she was holding it. We just thought how terribly clever. Surely her future achievements would make us proud of her.

What parents among us haven't envisioned our child reaching some glorified goal? Each child is special to us. We watch every motion and work it into some proud thought. We are sure the first words "mama" and "dada" have never been said quite so well by any other child. And so soon! We parents do well in this private world of pride and love.

In all honesty, now that the years have passed, I must admit Nancy was quite average and quite normal. She responded when she ought to and sometimes when I would rather she didn't. She would reach out for toys, hold them, then quickly loose interest and was off on to the next thing that took her fancy.

Nancy acquired a silver spoon from a doting relative and soon learned what it was for. She delighted in stirring vegetables in her bowl, then slopping them over the sides, making designs and swirls. The last she did somewhat artistically. But getting her to spoon up the conglomeration and put it into her mouth was another story. She continued to exercise her right to rebel.

My patience was tried. When it came to oatmeal, I

just about gave up. As fast as I spooned it in, her pink tongue thrust it out and down her chin where in clung like an old man's beard.

"There is nothing wrong with her," our doctor kept insisting. "She will eat when she is hungry."

Miraculously she did grow. And, she acquired a love for milk. Wonderful fresh, cold milk, with its protein, calcium and other elements her body needed for proper development. Thank goodness for her love of milk. That elixir of the gods was her saving grace in later years.

Although quite normal in her responses and growth the first year, she was slow to walk. She would pull herself up in the playpen or crib and walk around as she clung to the railings, but she just would not take the first step alone. Out on the floor, even with our encouragement, she would hold tightly to a chair or our hands, then slowly sink down when the support was removed. Possibly her legs weren't ready. They were spindly and long and we did not want to hurry her.

"Has she taken her first steps alone yet?" Friends and family kept asking.

"Not yet. She will any day, though." My answer was almost apologetic. Silly. Each child had his or her own personal time schedule. She would walk when she was ready.

Twelve months. Thirteen. Fourteen. Still no first step alone. Then one evening we sat on the living room floor playing with her. Nancy leaned over and grasped her father's bent knee. She pulled herself up to a standing position. We watched, hoping she wouldn't sink down again. She looked from Fred to me, opened her eyes wide and puckered her lips in a half kiss, half smile. Suddenly she stretched out both her arms. Without hesitation, she left the sturdy support of Fred's knee and came toward me. One step. Two steps. Then she fell.

"She did it!" I cried out.

We both leaned over and hugged her tightly. A loud squeal filled the room as she tried to release herself from our smothering affection.

In the days following, she tried again and again. A few more steps each time. Whenever she fell, she rolled around into a knee position like a runner in a race. Hands on the floor. Then up and away. A smile. A laugh. Excitement in her eyes. Now the world was hers. What places to explore! Kitchen cabinets. Waste baskets. Bookcases. So much to see and touch. Too much to stay with any one object for long. No time to put anything back. Forge ahead toward the next curiosity. Normal. Good. Our child was okay!

By sixteen months Nancy walked well. I wondered if her slowness had been because of her tall, slight build. Perhaps her back and legs had needed the extra time. I let it go at that.

From her first step onward, we watched Nancy's progress ourselves. Pediatricians weren't the "in" thing in those days. Our family doctor took charge of whatever care was needed. And little care appeared to be needed in the first few years except for the usual diphtheria, tetanus shots and vaccinations. The doctor visits were few and the reports always okay. She appeared to be developing normally.

There was no reason to think otherwise.

CHAPTER THIRTEEN

Horses and Angels

Sunrises. Sunsets. Our days came and went. Nancy had taken her first steps, eventually was weaned from her bottle, learned to speak her first words, tried to make us understand how she felt.

When Nancy was two, we moved into the "old house" my late grandfather had lived in. Situated on several acres, the house was just down the hill from where mom and pop lived. With the house and land came a brook, a pond, three deep wells, fields filled with daisies, buttercups and violets, three sugar maple trees, a crabapple tree, and granny's rhubarb and asparagus patches I later learned how to coax back into production.

With very little money, much hope and many plans, we began to rebuild the neglected, rotting New England Saltbox. The floors and ceilings sagged. The plumbing and wiring were about gone. The central air heater, resting on the dank dirt cellar floor, was rusted out. Everywhere we turned we saw work. Yet, each night I dropped off to sleep wanting morning to hurry and come so I could begin another day.

Because the house had been left empty for so many years and was in such a bad state, for the first several months we left Nancy with my mother during the day, until Fred could repair the floors and I could eliminate the mice.

We scraped floors and sanded woodwork, at least what we could save. We ripped out walls and tore up flooring that was too far gone, removed outside clapboards and replaced windows. Every job was done with the idea of saving the old that could not be replaced, the wide pine floorboards upstairs, authentic colonial paneled doors with latches, wainscoting in the dining room and wide granite front steps.

Nancy and I still found time for our peanut butter

and jelly sandwich picnics. We looked for buttercups and daisies in the fields beyond the house and usually ended up satisfied with fuzzy dandelions. Many afternoons we sat on the grass covered bridge over the brook that ran through the back of our property. We dangled our toes over the fieldstone edge, mine reaching the trickle of clear water beneath.

Nancy was up and down, exerting the typical energy of any two-year-old. She would finger her well-squeezed bunch of flowers, take a bite of her sandwich, then for a miraculous moment, sit still. One of those moments children have when the whole world rushes towards them and fills them with wonder and they are speechless.

Looking over at my child, I saw the beginnings of awareness in her blue eyes as she thrust the dandelions toward me and said, "See, mommy? Pretty!"

"Yes, darling," I answered. "Very pretty."

Those days spent in the golden fields were to sustain us in the years to come, just as our love for the sea would.

The times along the way I remember most were not the ones that burst with excitement and doings. Rather, they were the quiet moments when everything seemed to stop, all time compressed right then in a moment of understanding and truth. How often since I have gone back and tried to remember just such moments when my feelings cried out, *"God's in His Heaven and all's right with the world!"*

Memories of our little tea parties. Using her dolls' china cups, Nancy served silver tea made with hot water and sugar. My granny had taught mama and mama had taught me. Now I had the joy of teaching my own daughter.

Memories of her bedtime antics. Parading around in her p.j.s, she would giggle and laugh, then pounce on her bed and proceed to jump up and down. She'd pull the covers over her head, then giggle some more until I began an "off the top of my head" story, ending the day with, *"Now I lay me down to sleep."*

Of course our days were not always so tranquil. I certainly was not a perfect mother. Nancy was certainly not a perfect child. There were moments I wished I could float away on a cloud. The moments didn't last long, though.

And, of course, we had the doubts and differences natural to any family. There were constant trials to face and resolve. Two of Nancy's early trials had been to accept eating and learning to walk as necessary and even a bit enjoyable.

From there she went on to the other steps leading to the upper rungs of the ladder where grownups were. Learning what was and what was not. Learning what was allowed and what was not. Mostly, learning that dreams and desires did not always coincide with what could be. Since I kept no detailed journal of Nancy's development, I can't remember exactly when the wish presented itself. But present itself it did indeed.

"A horse daddy," she said one day as she leaned over the arm of his chair. With a big grin on her face she peered up into his eyes and asked, "Can I have a horse?"

A normal enough request for a four-year-old. Most children's books pictured the sleek animals galloping into the wind. The words may have read, *"A horse. Jane sees a horse. Jane rides the horse."* The primer should have helped us not so affluent parents by adding, *"Horses eat. They eat a lot. And often they need shelter from the cold. A barn costs money. Lots of money."*

"Daddy?" she asked again, this time rumpling his paper and placing herself squarely in front of him.

Fred dropped his paper and cupped her pleading face in his hands. "Honey, I wish you could have one."

"But daddy, you had horses when you were a little boy."

So he had. On the farm in Maine. They were not a luxury though. They had earned their keep by pulling the plow and harrow. Fred tried to explain. Nancy listened, pouted, then left his side. I watched her go outside to her doll carriage parked under the sugar maple tree. She picked up her doll and cradled it in her arms.

No more was said about horses for a long time afterward. We were busy putting our money and energy into rebuilding. How could we possibly buy a horse, much less provide it food and shelter? We couldn't. So that ended the matter right there. Or so we thought.

Nancy appeared to be growing straight and her appetite began to pick up a bit. For that I was grateful, although, she still had no desire for a variety of vegetables. It never occurred to me to run my fingers down her spine to check if she was really growing straight. I simply assumed she was. No doctor ever mentioned otherwise.

As we watch our children grow straight in body, we also pray they will grow straight in spirit. Inevitably questions come up which we parents are expected to have all the answers to. How do we explain something that we, ourselves, cannot put into words? We wait for the right moment when, in a flash of truth, our children become aware of the goodness and intensity of life and the existence of the living God. By reflecting our own feelings, he or she knows instinctively. So we wait.

One summer evening we were sitting on the blue stone front step listening to crickets out on the lawn and frogs down in the pond. As we leaned back, breathing in the scent of early summer, fireflies appeared all around us and seemed to be trying to out do the stars in the sky.

Nancy jumped up and ran after one as it lit up over the tulip bed near the old cellar wall. She quickly ran back to us and sat down between her father and me, leaning her head on my arm.

"There must be a God," she said.

"Oh? Why?" I asked.

"You and daddy can't make fireflies light up, can you?

"No..."

"Besides, my Guardian Angel needs Him to tell her what to do. I do have one, right?"

"I'm sure you do," I said.

"With two Angel Wings?"

"Of course. With two Angel Wings. How else could she fly?"

"Oh, good."

Nancy rubbed her face in the softness of my sweater as the three of us sat safe and secure in our own little world.

CHAPTER FOURTEEN

My Crooked Little Girl

During her first five years Nancy had the usual childhood colds, cuts and scrapes. Thankfully, nothing more. Chicken pox popped up before the start of school. She was miserable, but recovered with no major scars.

Parenthood was certainly not a cinch. As a mother, I still felt not so storybook capable. I picked up, scrubbed up, and wiped off. I got weary and impatient sometimes. Although idealistic poetry would have you believe it, becoming a mother didn't suddenly turn one into a tireless saint. Motherhood could be physically exhausting at times, but it more often than not brought wonderful gifts.

Life was progressing true to our dreams, even with the occasional disappointments and difficult days. What family didn't have them? We were quite normal. Tempers and tears had their place amongst the smiles and laughter. Nancy was growing tall and slim like her dad and his mother. The Webster build. I would smile and nod.

Our house remodeling progressed. With new plumbing, wiring, heating and a modern kitchen finished, we moved on to redo one half of the downstairs into a pine-paneled living room with a huge fireplace. I learned how to paper and paint, make braided rugs and canned hundreds of jars of vegetables.

A pile of red brick lay heaped beside the drive, waiting to be used. By now we three were veterans at maneuvering around lumber, shingles, piping and other assorted building materials. So what was a pile of bricks to worry about?

About that time, the first of two accidents happened. Neither one needed recording. They were ones not likely to be forgotten.

One warm summer day I stood in our kitchen, picking over a basket of blueberries Nancy and I had gathered from the field across the street. Remembering how mama had taught me, I picked over the blueberries by rolling them across a clean dishtowel, separating the leaves and bad berries by pushing them to the side, then rolling the good berries down off the countertop and into my colander.

I stood next to the freshly painted white cabinets with their black antique hinges, occasionally looking out the back entry door to the yard where Nancy played under the sugar maple tree. With its branches spread wide over the lawn, it was her favorite spot to play. Suddenly, in a burst of energy, she ran from the maple tree down the path to the barn cellar. She stopped, turned, and started back up. Halfway to the tree she stumbled and fell.

One scream. Nothing more.

I dropped the colander on the countertop and flew out the screen door to where Nancy lay face down, her forehead smashed on the corner of a brick. As I gently picked her up, blood streamed from the gash just below her hairline. Her body lay rigid in my arms. Her breathing had nearly stopped. Holding her, I could feel her warm blood spilling onto my blouse and arms. Quickly I carried her back into the kitchen and began to douse her face and neck with cold water. I tapped her cheeks, then held her face in the palms of my hands.

"Cry! Do something!"

Her eyes twitched. She refocused them in one quick jerk from the ceiling to me.

"Mommy!" She reached her arms out and wrapped them tightly around my neck. The whole room filled with her sobs.

I grabbed the phone and called my mother. Moments later she pulled into the yard. What would we do without our mothers and doctors? I bundled Nancy into the car and held a cold wet cloth to her forehead while my mother drove us to our doctor's office. Family doctors were usually readily available in those days, and unhurried. No rush in. No rush out. Dr. Carolyn knew us well and could spot trouble almost before it began. If we needed to talk, he took the time. Such comfort.

Nancy's sobs were exhausted gulps by the time I carried her into the familiar office.

"Well now, what have we done?" Our doctor held out his strong arms and took her from me. He cleaned and dressed the wound, all the while speaking in a soothing tone of voice, as much for me as for Nancy. She started to tell her tale and by the time he finished, he had her story down pat. Nancy's love and respect for good doctors was firmly planted that day. Our doctor's gentle hands and his words of assurance combined to set us both at ease.

He sent us home with pats on the shoulders and the parting words, "Take it easy, Nancy. Don't try to smash any more bricks."

To me he added, "I believe she will be just fine. However, I would advise you call me if there is any change."

My faith in him was unshakable. This same kind of faith I would transfer to another doctor years later when we placed Nancy's whole future in his hands.

Not long after the first accident, the second occurred. Although these types of accidents may appear far removed from the development of her spine, they did have significance. Both reinforced her love and trust for the medical profession.

That fall we three drove to the Berkshire Mountains for a long weekend. The horizon was ablaze with reds, yellows and oranges. We enjoyed warm, golden Indian Summer days and crisp clear nights, just like the first Indian Summer days of our marriage. Nancy sensed our hunger to take in every aspect of fall's breathtaking finale.

At one point, after standing on the roadside to look across the gentle mountain slopes, we hurried back to our car. In haste, I flung the door open. Nancy was right behind me and rushed headlong into it. There was no gash this time, just a bruised indentation.

"Shhh... Shhh... It will be okay..." I brushed her hair back and kissed her forehead. How careless, I thought. How stupidly careless of me. One quick second was all it took. I hugged Nancy tight, trying to release my feelings of guilt as I comforted her. She clung to my arms, her head resting on my shoulder as I whispered softly to her. Gradually her tears lessened. We went on our way, sure everything was all right.

Two days later I watched Nancy run to greet Fred as he returned home from work.

"Daddy! Daddy!"

As she flung out her arms he caught her up and swung her around, her hands clasped tightly around his neck. He stopped, looked at her for a moment, then carried her into the house.

Without answering my "hi" he turned Nancy's face toward me and cupped her chin in his palm.

"Didn't you notice her eye?"

"Oh, no..." I said. "She was okay a little while ago. She's been playing while I was busy in the kitchen. Oh, God, no!"

I stared at Nancy's face. Her left eye was turned in toward her nose. I felt sick to my stomach. It had to be the bang on her forehead. The car door. It was my fault. I reached over to take her, but Fred held Nancy tight in his one arm and stretched his other arm out to restrain me.

"Take it easy, now." His controlled manner had a way of bringing me into check.

That night, lying in bed, I kept saying to myself, "What have I done?"

It was all my fault. Gradually I quelled my guilt with rationalization. Children were always having little accidents. Never the less, I knew we had to do something about it.

Happenings come in threes, I've heard. That Nancy's crooked eye was to be the first of three crookeds never entered my mind. I had no inkling that one day I would lovingly call Nancy my crooked little girl. Crooked eye. Crooked teeth. Crooked spine. All three would need medical supervision and correction.

Even at five years old, little girls could be vain. Nancy wanted straight eyes, so it was no problem to convince her to wear the corrective patch, do the necessary eye exercises and wear her metal rimmed glasses. Doctors at Massachusetts General Eye Clinic saw her through this period and brought one fact home to me. A cooperative relationship between patient and doctor was the key to successful results. All three crooked and their correction made me positive that such teamwork could work miracles.

CHAPTER FIFTEEN

The Dreaded Word

I was not concerned with miracles in those early days. More down to earth things were about to happen. Nancy started school. On her first day I watched my child walk away from me, her light brown hair parted on the left and brushed to the sides with a red ribbon catching it near the top. Her metal rimmed glasses slipped down her nose and she pushed them back into place. She turned to me and waved.

"Bye, mom!"

She had never called me that before. The hand I just let go of had never held that of a teacher's either. Dressed in her starched cotton dress and wool cardigan sweater, Nancy entered her first grade class room, joining all the other well-scrubbed youngsters. I swallowed hard and knew it was time to leave.

On the third day a call came from the school nurse. Nancy was not feeling well and she requested I come down and pick Nancy up. On the way to Dr. Carolyn's, she the threw up all over herself and the front seat.

"Fever? Flu?" I asked the doctor.

"No," came his answer.

"Nerves?"

"No. Not really. Just an emotional adjustment many children go through."

Nancy overcame her initial shyness, soon adjusting to the routine, her teacher, and the other children. The days following, we said goodbye at our front door. Morning sun filtering through the mist in the field across the street filled our doorway, making the new colonial door appear whiter. Kneeling down on one of the blue stone front steps, I kissed Nancy's cheek and pushed back a wisp of hair. After turning her around for a last inspection, I hugged her tight.

"Off you go!"

She skipped as far as the gate of the split rail fence. Once on the street, she broke into a run toward the top of the hill, her lunch pail swinging back and forth on her arm. Nancy's greatest concern was that she might miss her bus. What greater concern should a six-year-old have?

She made friends, brought them home to play, studied her lessons and occasionally brought up the subject of horses. She didn't beg. She just talked. We always listened.

Maybe someday, I thought. Maybe.

In a child's way, though, she already had her horse. The gate of our split rail fence had posts just right for holding the reins. The top rail, padded with an old doll blanket, made a good saddle.

"Giddy up!" she called out. "Ride like lightning! Giddy up like thunder!" She leaned forward to pat the post, then straightened when she pretended her horse broke into a canter, her feet firmly set on the middle rail, her stirrups.

Nearby, I listened to her child's play while I sat in the rope swing hanging from our horse chestnut tree. Nancy brought her pretend horse to a halt by pulling hard on the reins, then swung her leg over the railing to dismount, off to some other play.

During the fall of her first school year, Nancy caught a cold accompanied by a severe sore throat. She finally got rid of it, then promptly got sick again. Her school doctor advised having her tonsils removed. In 1953 tonsillectomies were just another routine surgery, although today tonsils are considered protection to the body and are removed only if absolutely necessary.

We consulted Dr. Carolyn, who also advised surgery. We agreed.

Unfortunately, hospitals were severely over crowded, many with polio patients, the crippling disease increasing at alarming rates. The hospital Nancy had been born in had no room for her. Another small hospital nearby did, and arrangements were made.

Nancy did not like the idea of staying in the hospital overnight, but when the time came she didn't balk. She went quietly with the nurse, who undressed her, put her in a hospital gown and settled her in bed.

Later, I patched some facts together. There may

never be a sure answer. Human curiosity, however, keeps searching out of pure need.

Before Nancy's arrival, her hospital room had sheltered several polio patients. One wall of her room was a glass floor to ceiling window. On the other side a long row of hospital beds still held some of the less severe polio cases.

I'm sure every precaution was taken, every confirmed case put immediately into isolation. This was a good hospital. Not one of us in 1953 could ever imagine the nightmare just beginning. Every hospital in New England, in fact in all of America, was to face increasing polio cases in 1954 and epidemic proportions in 1955 and 1956. With fever, sore muscles, intense pain, stiffness, and finally paralysis, it became one of the most feared diseases of our time.

My mind goes back vividly to the day I read through reports written by Dr. Paul Harrington of Houston, Texas, who developed and perfected the rod and fusion method for correcting spinal curvature. He listed three possible causes of scoliosis (curvature of the spine). First, idiopathic (having no know cause) accounting for over 60% of the cases, second, post-poliomyelitic, accounting for 31%, and third, congenital, accounting for the remaining 9%.

Nancy was officially listed under the idiopathic category. She had been born healthy and not treated for polio. I, being a mother, was not satisfied with the unknown category. Especially when my mind goes back to that green hospital room with the glass windows and the whispered words, *polio.*

Nancy said "ahh" that day as the nurse tucked her into her hospital bed. She was taken to the operating room and awoke several hours later minus her tonsils and adenoids. We took her home the next day and promptly marked the whole episode as a normal step in growing up.

CHAPTER SIXTEEN

Measles

My questions and searching went on. In retrospect, however, the seriousness and humor of life always seemed to mingle. Thank goodness life doesn't go all in one vain, good or bad.

In thinking back, I now realize there are many ways we can endear ourselves to relatives and friends. And, there are ways we can, without even trying, encourage alienation.

February 1955. We looked forward to our first trip south. Florida was a magical place we had seen only in travel brochures and magazines. We'd just been through another summer and fall of ever increasing new polio cases. Now that the New England weather was well set in with ice and snow, we sat by our new brick fireplace and dreamed of warm sunshine, soft breezes and sandy beaches. Fred's carpentry work had slowed and he welcomed the chance to get away from the freezing winds that cracked his hands and frost bit his nose. We were more than ready to head straight down U.S. # 1.

Nancy was a great help in packing. "Can I take this? And this?" she asked, laying out her best summer clothes beside her swimsuit and schoolbooks. We had the okay from her teacher, who had given Nancy enough assignments to last the several weeks we planned to stay in Florida.

"Nancy is up to date in all her studies," her teacher told me. "And with her books, I am sure she can work along by herself." In second grade, Nancy was familiar with what was expected of her.

Suitcases bulging and cameras ready, we were all set to go. Fred's Aunt Kate, who lived with us now, and Nancy rode in the back seat. Seventy-five years versus seven. What separated them in age, they made up for in enthusiasm.

Fred and I were glad to get away too. Along with the endless thought of polio, there was another threat in Nancy's classroom. Measles.

"Paul just came down with them," Nancy said to us when we were part way down the East Coast.

"With what?" I asked, my mind taken up with the thoughts of sun, sand and beaches ahead of us.

"With measles, mom!"

"Measles? Paul? Just what we need. Poor Paul. I'm glad we left when we did. You don't sit near him in class, do you?"

"Not exactly..."

At that moment we noticed something that caught our attention and left the subject behind. Or so we thought.

We stopped for a few days in Asbury Park and stayed at the Rexmere Hotel. Aunt Kate often wintered there with her cousins who owned and operated it. How welcoming, the hominess of the big rambling building. We drank morning coffee in the huge kitchen, ate lunch and dinner in the main dining room, sitting amidst the older guests. Later we joined them for Bingo. Nancy had the run of the place, mingling with everyone.

On our third day there her energy seemed to wane. We walked down to the fishing pier to watch pelicans strut around. Nancy fussed at my suggestion to walk to the end.

"I don't want to." She made a funny face at me.

I didn't argue. Perhaps she was tired from all the excitement. A good night's sleep would fix her up.

The next morning the three of us left for Miami. Aunt Kate wanted to stay on and visit with her cousins. We waved goodbye to our silver haired friends standing on the wide wooden porch steps. We were off.

Nancy laid down in the back seat, quite unusual for her. So far she had kept up with her assignments, but now she pushed the books aside and they lay on the floor beside her. She curled up on the seat and fell asleep, her light brown pigtails flopping over the pillow, her sandaled feet hanging over the edge.

In Miami we bypassed the lushness of Collins Avenue. Our budget wouldn't withstand the pressure. Instead, we rented a cabin style motel room located on busy

Biscayne Boulevard. We were equidistant from the ocean to the east and Fred's brother, Dick, to the west.

The next day Dick and his wife Bette took us for a sight seeing drive along the beach. Nancy and her cousin Marilyn were getting aquatinted, sitting in the front seat between Dick and Bette. As we drove along enjoying the beach scenery, Nancy began to sniffle.

"She'd better ride back here with us if she's catching another cold. No need for Marilyn to catch it," I commented.

"She's okay," Dick answered. "What's a little cold?"

That night at the motel Nancy became restless. She sneezed a few times and felt hot when I touched her forehead. An aspirin, some sleep, and she would be better in the morning.

When she awakened, she was fussy and her forehead was hotter than the previous evening. As the day progressed, she became worse. We called a doctor at a clinic close by and were given an appointment almost immediately.

"Ah hah," he said. "Mmm..."

"What is it? What is wrong with her?"

"Measles."

"Measles? Oh, no! She can't have them on our only trip to Florida!"

"Well, she does."

"The real kind?"

"The real kind," he repeated.

The next few days seemed to run together. Night into day. Day into night. There, in that small motel room, we were in a world of our own. Isolated. I remember the oldness of it against the newness of the lush beach hotels we had seen only a few days earlier. Nancy lay on a single bed pushed up against one wall. Our twin beds were on the other side of the rough plastered room.

I slept very little; conscious of Nancy's fevered breathing. I sponged her forehead and fluffed her pillow, turning it every hour so the cool side was to her face.

The next day I walked up to the office. "Please, may I have fresh sheets each day and extra ice water? My child is very sick."

They complied with my requests with cool politeness. I don't think they liked the idea of a measles case in one of their units. It certainly wouldn't do much for business if the other guests knew.

Because the motel had no restaurant, Fred and I took turns going to a drugstore three blocks away for meals. Not exactly my idea of a romantic stay on Miami Beach, eating 85 cent lunches sitting on a drugstore stool. We made it though. I ordered hot soup and took it back to Nancy.

By the next night she was delirious. She mumbled and jumbled her words together. I couldn't understand a thing she said, but I hoped this was the peak of the illness. I sponged her with alcohol and sat holding her as she flung out her arms.

"It's okay, honey. Quiet now. It's all right. Mommy is here."

Finally, toward morning, she quieted and fell into an exhausted sleep. Hours later, with my eyelids stuck together, I heard her weak voice.

"Mom. Mom."

I groped my way over to Nancy and knelt down.

"I'm hungry, mom," she said, smiling up at me for the first time in days.

"Thank God." I hugged her to me. "We'll have to see what we can do about that."

Nancy had survived a severe case of measles. In reading about the causes of scoliosis, the questions came again. Could this have been part of the cause? At the time, though, my only concern, other than Nancy's recovery, was Marilyn. Would she get them too?

She did, unfortunately. But recovered in her own good time.

CHAPTER SEVENTEEN

Epidemic

The summers of 1955 and 1956 prompted mixed emotions in every American. The good and bad, to the limit of our endurance. We could sum them up in two phrases: "Polio rising to epidemic proportions" and "Salk discovers polio vaccine." The second should have canceled out the first, but the two ran parallel for some time.

When the news broke in 1955, we heard it from all directions at once. Radio, television, newspapers, friends, clerks in stores, people on the street.

"The vaccine! They've got the vaccine!" everyone was saying. "Our children will be safe now!"

In our relief we didn't think about time, the interval between the discovery and the availability of the vaccine. Time. That precious intangible we possess, yet do not possess. In one second the whole future can be spelled out. None of us knew anything for sure.

In the beginning of those frightening, yet hopeful days, production of the vaccine was hurried along as quickly as possible. I envied those receiving it. Their awful wait was over. How short lived my envy was. Of the first people to receive the vaccine, some contracted crippling polio. I was confused and angry. Had medical science been too hasty in trying to push the vaccine before it was proven completely safe?

Word finally came. The basic vaccine was all right. Fault lay in the production. Some of the first batches contained live polio virus. The wait began again.

During the waiting we tried not to think about polio.

"Mom?" Nancy begged more than once during the hot summer of 1955. "Can we go swimming down in the pool in the park?"

"Not today," I answered, smoothing back her light

brown hair.

"When then?" she continued.

"I don't know darling. I just don't know."

A thought came to me. Why not build a little swimming pool for Nancy and her friends? It couldn't be that hard. If I could put in 150 feet of split rail fence, certainly I could figure this out.

Nancy and I selected a spot just on the other side of the horse chestnut tree and, with a lightened heart, I set to work. Following my rough outline in the grass, Fred helped me dig a hole two feet deep. We ended up with an area about ten feet long and five feet wide. Plenty of room for several little girls to splash around in.

Fred brought home wire mesh, laying it along the bottom and sides for me. I mixed cement by hand in my wheel barrow, bag after bag, adding in sand and water, then pouring it in until the bottom and sides were covered with several inches. I finished the top edges with good sized, smooth rocks and cemented them together. After several days of "curing" I hauled out a long hose and began filling my creation.

Nancy was thrilled and soon invited several of her playmates to try it out. While Nancy and her friends played in the pool, I stayed nearby digging in the garden, or working in the yard, always keeping my eye on them.

Nancy turned eight in July. One day, soon after her birthday, she came to me.

"Mom? Feel."

She placed my hand on her forehead. It was hot and her eyes looked glassy. Taking her hand, I led her up the steep, narrow stairs to Fred's and my room with the big double bed. There I undressed her and she slid between cool white sheets.

"I hurt mom. I hurt."

"Where do you hurt?" I waited for her answer with mounting panic.

"Right here." She raised her hand and touched her neck.

Her neck? Not her neck! I wouldn't let the word polio enter our world. In the bathroom I rinsed the thermometer off under cold water, shook it down, then went back to put it under Nancy's tongue. I rushed downstairs to call Dr. Carolyn. His nurse told me he was unavailable and she would have him call back as soon as he could.

"My neck hurts so much!" Nancy cried with I returned to remove the thermometer. It had shot up alarmingly high.

"Everything will be all right." I kissed her forehead, then slipped into the hall, sitting on the top step. I gazed down the steep stairway to the white colonial front door which still stood open in my haste to get Nancy into bed. Outside was a perfect summer day. I could see the horse chestnut tree and split rail beyond.

Go like lighting! Ride like thunder! I imagined my child sitting again on the cedar gate, calling out to her pretend horse.

"Oh, no..." I cried silent tears, burying my face in my hands.

The shrill ringing of the telephone jolted me back to reality. I ran down the stairs two at a time. Dr. Carolyn was too busy to come. Just where did she hurt? Could she walk, move her head and arms? Could she swallow? I answered each of his questions. Then there was silence.

"Is it..." The words were too painful to finish.

He knew me well and read my thoughts. "Polio?"

"Yes. Is it?" I asked.

His answer came back firm and seemingly assured.

"No."

"What then?" I asked.

"From your description of all her symptoms, I'd say, mumps."

"Mumps?"

"Yes, mumps. But keep me informed if there is any change whatsoever."

He instructed me on care and with overwhelming relief, I hung up the phone.

Back in my room, I rushed past the bed where Nancy lay, trying to hide my tears as I brushed them away. There I stood, looking out through the small paned window down to the lawn and crabapple tree. Wild crabapples were just beginning to ripen. Nancy and I would pick them in the fall. We'd wash and put them into a boiling pot on the stove. There would be crabapple jelly next winter; jars and jars of it stored on preserve shelves in the cellar. Winter would come soon and with it a tapering off of new polio cases. Maybe by then the vaccine would be available to everyone.

"Mom?" Nancy called out to me.

"Yes, darling," I answered. "Everything is going to be okay. I was just looking at the beautiful crop of crabapples we are going to have."

By the summer of 1956 we dreaded even going to the store. We all faced the fact that there was no security anywhere. More and more people came down with fever and pain that defined the remainder of their lives. In one word, paralysis. Newspapers didn't spell it out in exact letters - *EPIDEMIC*. They simply advised caution, to stay away from the beach, or any crowded place.

We were lucky. We had land, fresh air and sun-shine. Nancy now had her own little swimming pool. We could roam the fields across the street from the old house and gather blueberries. There were buttercups and dandelions to pick. Robins and bluebirds nested and searched for food. Flying about in the scrub pine and maples along the pasture's edge, I wondered if they were any more secure in their world?

"Here, Mom!" Nancy called out to me. "Here's a four-leaf clover!"

In our excitement, we both reached down, only to find it had the usual three leaves. We laughed and picked it up anyway.

I wonder, now, if perhaps we were a bit selfish in our isolation. Just twenty miles away in Boston, tenements housed family after family with the same desires for life. Yet they were trapped in the hot, stale air, compressed into dark hallways and tiny apartments. They walked along steaming sidewalks. Compression, exposure, then the inevitable infection.

That same summer Aunt Kate became ill and needed to have her gall bladder removed. She was admitted to Massachusetts General Hospital in Boston. The night I checked her in she was placed in an examining room, one of many such rooms lining both sides of a long hallway. Walking down that hall, it was hard not to notice how many doors were closed with posted signs - *POLIO?* That word and question mark remain in my mind to this day. A shudder went through me as I walked out to Nancy and her dad waiting in the car.

Each day we drove in to visit Aunt Kate. Each day I left Nancy in the car with her dad. Each day I saw the polio signs. I was relieved when Aunt Kate was well enough to come home.

Soon, too soon afterward, a friend of ours came down with fever that raked his body. The news came. Norman was completely paralyzed and in an iron lung. I grasped Nancy and held her tight. No, not us. Not our family. Not our friends. Not anyone else. We'd all had enough...

During the late summer of 1956, Nancy and I kept busy picking blueberries in the fields across the street. Each afternoon we tied our wicker baskets around our waists, walking further into the fields in hopes of finding the plumpest berries. Nancy delighted in being the first to find a new bush filled with ripe berries. It was one of the few things I knew would take her mind, as well as mine, away from having to stay so close to home. As we walked, we made sure to give the red ant hills a wide berth. Getting stung was not something we wanted to experience.

Each day, after blueberry picking, I spread a cloth on the kitchen table and picked through the berries. Nancy pulled her chair close to mine, playing happily with one of her dolls, every once in a while sneaking a berry or two to munch on. We ended up picking enough berries for me to can over 100 jars, ready to store in the cellar.

Summer had finally passed. The briskness of the days signified its end. Nancy and I gathered crabapples. We clambered along stone walls to pluck wild grapes hanging in bunches above us. We picked the last of the tomatoes and cucumbers. All these we took to the kitchen and soon we were enjoying the familiar aroma of sweet spices as pots bubbled with jellies and piccalilli in the making.

Nancy started fourth grade. Several weeks into the new school year she brought home the announcement that her class was scheduled to receive the new polio vaccine. My faith was sprinkled with fear at the memory of those first batches. If the mistake had occurred once, couldn't it again?

The day of her vaccine shot she came home favoring her arm. "It hurts," she said, dropping her books onto the dining room table. "But, guess what? Miss Fisk let us do whatever we wanted after we got our shots."

I noticed where the needle had gone in leaving a tiny red spot. "Oh? And what did you do?"

"I colored. Here. See?" Nancy pulled a paper from her books and laid it down. She had colored a wild, beautiful horse cantering, his mane flowing in the wind.

"Mom, someday, do you think..."

"Think what?"

"Do you think I could have a horse like him some-day? Or, at least ride one?"

She hadn't forgotten her dream. Perhaps we could let her try riding. There were stables not too far away. Maybe next week we could take a drive and inquire about riding lessons.

Almost overnight, the cold of late fall came and with it the planning ahead to the holidays. A busy time. No time to begin horseback riding. Halloween. Thanksgiving. Christmas.

Nancy had her second polio shot and came through like a veteran.

"Had another shot today, mom," she called out to me in the kitchen.

"Good." I let an apple skin curl down under my peeler and fall into the colander.

"Apple pie for supper?" Nancy now stood beside me snitching a few slices from the bowl on the counter.

I leaned over, kissed the top of her head, then tapped her hand. "No more now or there won't be any apples left for our pie."

Later that evening, sitting in front of our fireplace, I watched the logs burn down to a deep glow. Fred sat in his chair, his head behind the paper. Nancy was up in her room studying. Our world was secure. With the threat of polio over for us, what could possibly mar our lives?

Sitting on the footstool, I touched the log with the poker. Hopes. Dreams. The future. Someday our child would be grown and married and it would again be just the two of us. I looked over at Fred as he came out from behind his paper.

"Where's Nancy?"

"In her room studying."

"Oh." He leaned forward. As he looked at the fire I felt that his thoughts must have been running alongside mine. This was what life was all about. A home. The warmth of being comfortable together. And having a child. What greater fulfillment could anyone seek?

Suddenly I heard hurried steps on the stairs. Nancy peeked her head around the corner. "Mom, can I have another piece of apple pie?" She swung herself into the room and I felt the completeness of our lives.

"Good idea. Another piece of apple pie," Fred said, dropping his paper in a heap on the floor.

CHAPTER EIGHTEEN

Deciding on the Big Move

Christmas came with its flourish of doings and its dazzling beauty. Snow crunched outside, logs crackled inside, family and friends feasted together. What a Christmas! There would be no dreaded fear of polio during the coming summer. We would be able to walk the dusty streets of Boston or swim at the park pool in town if we wished. The threat of polio was over.

When the last bit of tinsel had been put away we felt the usual after holiday let-down. One evening in January, Fred set up the movie projector and we watched time slip back to our trip to Florida two winters before.

I remembered how, on our way home, we had stopped briefly for one last look at the ocean. Not bothering to take off my loafers, I had run across the beach to the edge of the water. On my way back to the car, I felt sand packed in around my toes. I slipped my shoes off, dumping the tiny grains.

"We'll be back, Nancy. We'll be back. That's what they say about getting sand in your shoes."

"Really, mom?" Nancy dug her feet down deep. Her sandals filled with fine white grains. She slipped them off and dumped the sand. "That's to make sure," she said with a giggle.

What we wouldn't give now for that sun and sand.

"Let's go to Florida again," Fred said when the last roll of film ran off.

"Could we, daddy?"

It was a wild idea, but the thought of sunshine and warm sandy beaches excited me too.

"Why not pack up and go for the rest of the winter?" Fred continued.

"Yes, daddy, let's. Mom?"

Fred would have to find work. Nancy would have to

go to school. That night we left the subject hanging in midair.

When Fred came home from work the next day, he laid his hammer and saw down on the radiator in the kitchen as he had been doing ever since the January freeze set in.

"What about it?" How soon can you be ready?"

"You mean it, daddy?" Nancy pulled on his arm and took his cracked and split hands in hers.

My first question was, "What about Aunt Kate?"

Fred, always the pragmatist, answered, "She'll be fine. She's comfortable in her little apartment and with her own phone your mother can check on her every couple of days."

Nancy piped in, "And I can play with Marilyn and maybe ride horses?"

"Well, I think we can be packed in a few days," I answered.

"Oh, goody, goody!" Nancy grabbed my hand, jumping up and down.

That evening, we sat looking over maps in front of the log fire in the living room.

"It's settled then. We'll leave as soon as you're packed."

"Oh, daddy. Oh, mommy. Wait until I tell the kids at school!"

"Off to bed with you." I gave her a gentle tap and sent her on her way.

Later, when the house was quiet, I stood looking down at the last bit of embers. What a winter to remember. It would be good for all three of us. Little did I know that from that moment on our lives were to change completely.

To leave New England for good never entered our minds nor Nancy's. We were merely preparing for a few months stay in Florida. Then we would be back home, as usual. The next day or two we could scarcely hold in our excitement.

"I wonder what the kids down there are like," Nancy asked as she handed me several pairs of her shorts to pack.

"I guess they'll be like kids anywhere else." I folded and pressed several more tops down into her suitcase.

Outside the sky was gray and frosty, but I could barely see it through the layer of ice that clung to the inside of the storm window. Touching the radiator, I closed my eyes in anticipation. Anticipation of the weeks of warm sunshine ahead.

The next day we started off, with winter's cold and gray trying to follow us. Although we gradually left the ice-slicked highways behind, it was three more days before we saw a break in the gray skies.

Moments after passing the Florida welcoming station, as if to signal our arrival, the clouds parted and the sun reached down, touching the trees, road and car. Nancy reached out as if to capture the golden rays in her fists.

The following weeks were filled with sunshine, sandy beaches and Nancy's walks to school and back from the apartment we rented. She loved her teacher, quickly made new friends and soon became one of the best students in her class. Not only did she keep up with her new class, but also with her books and assignments from home. We laughingly called it her double dose of school.

With south Florida in a building boom, Fred easily found work with his brother Dick. Fred's work in the warm Florida sunshine quickly tanned him and healed his cracked and sore hands.

One evening we sat on the apartment steps looking up at the sky filled with fluffy clouds so low we could almost touch them.

"Let's move down," Fred said.

"You mean forever?" Nancy leaned against his arm.

"I'd like to." He gave her a bear hug.

When she broke away from him he yanked at her pigtails.

"Oh, daddy, you're just fooling."

He wasn't though. Each weekend we spent with Dick, Bette and Marilyn. While the girls played happily together, we tossed back and forth the idea of making the move permanent. Dick and Bette both encouraged us in the decision, giving us all the positives of living in Florida. The more we talked, the more convinced we were to make the move.

One afternoon, I sat down and wrote my mother a

letter, wanting to try and explain to her what we were thinking about doing. She immediately answered back. Her thoughts were clear. We were foolish to even think about moving. How could we leave her and pop? How could we leave the "old house" after all the work we had put into remodeling? We were foolish, just foolish.

From then on the letters flowed back and forth, her displeasure growing with each letter she wrote. I kept trying to assure mama that she would not be loosing us, that I would write every day, Nancy and I could visit them each summer, and they could come south and stay with us during the winter.

Fred and I talked and talked about what we should do with the old house. Sell it? Rent it? In my heart I knew I didn't want to sell it. I ached with the thought of leaving it, but if we sold it we would have a clean start with our new life in Florida. If we kept it and rented there would be the constant worry of upkeep, collecting rent, and continuing repairs.

I began to feel as if I didn't know my own mind. I kept going in circles with my thoughts, trying so hard to think of everything and everyone, wanting to do what was best for all concerned. How had this all become so complicated?

Despite mama's objections, we continued formulating our plans and finalized our decision. For Fred, the thought of working through another icy winter, hoping for enough carpentry work, knowing his hands would split open from the frigid temperatures, was too much. Dick lined up a job for Fred and we felt confident we were making the right move.

We called a real estate agent back home and put the "old house" up for sale. We went house hunting and found what we wanted in a new neighborhood several blocks from elementary and high schools for Nancy and only two miles from Dick and Bette. We put money into escrow and were promised the house would be finished by the time we returned.

One evening I read over a letter Nancy was writing to mom and pop. I envied her in how uncomplicated her life was.

March 3, 1957

Dear Nanna and Grampa,

I am having a good time in Fla. We went to the beach yesterday. We had fun. It was to cold to go swimming. But I went in once. We have bought a pretty house. It is right near a school to. We might go and see how they are doing on it. Marilyn came over last night and we played with her papper dolls. Mommy and daddy washed the car this morning and I helped them. I walk to school from our apt. We go from 830 to 300. We have found a park and mommy takes me there. I have gone on 2 pony rides. One was fast and the other one slow. How is Sandra and Susan and all the gang? I miss them very much. I miss you and grampa very much to. Why don't you and grampa come down here and live? Its very nice. Mommy said she is going too like it very much. I like it to.

Love,
Nancy

April 1, we headed back north. I dreaded returning home and talking to mom and pop in person. I knew it was going to be one of the hardest things I had ever done. I sat with them one afternoon and tried to explain it all again, but they still could not understand. The same questions came, fast and furious. How could we leave them? How could we leave the "old house?" How could we move so far away? For every positive I presented, they had a negative.

Tired and discouraged, I left them and walked down the hill. I thought about pop. Even though he had always wanted to live in Florida, he had never made the decision to move. I wondered how much of their displeasure was envy, or were they really just trying to keep us close? Fred and I had many more discussions with them, trying to assure them we believed we were doing what was best for us, and they could come and stay with us during the winter months for as long as they wanted.

I felt as if I was being pulled in two different directions. I started asking myself, *were we doing the right thing?* I wanted to do what was best for Fred, always trying to be a loving and supportive wife. On the other hand, I had always tried to be a respectful and loving daughter. Mom and pop continued to try and talk us out of the move, but we had made our decision. There was no turning back.

Nancy returned to Bird School and finished out her school year. We started picking through and weeding out every unnecessary item, packing what we could, and gave the rest away, including Fred's snow skis, Nancy's sled, and my 100 jars of canned blueberries.

On our last morning I walked upstairs to Nancy's empty bedroom, sat down on the floor and cried. Seven years of work and love had been built into every corner of this old house. The question came again, *how could we leave it?* In this very room night after night I had tucked Nancy in bed and listened to her prayers. We had measured her height on the door casing; the black pencil marks still visible. I ran my fingers over the wide pine board floor, clean and shiny with gray paint.

"Mom? Mom?" Suddenly Nancy's voice came from the bottom of the stairs. With a familiar clumping up the steep steps, she called out, "Daddy needs you!"

By the time she reached the doorway I was on my feet, the tears wiped away.

"Okay." I took her hand and we both went downstairs together.

Outside I helped load our most treasured possessions into the U Haul that would be hitched to the back of my car. Skipping past us, Nancy settled herself for a moment in her rope swing, then leapt off, letting the empty wood seat swing back and forth in the air. She rushed toward the split rail fence, grasped the top rail and hobbled the whole length to the drive in an uneven fashion, her right foot on the first rail, her left foot on the ground. She sang, "We're moving to Miami, Miami, Miami..."

Fred left first in an old black van filled to overflowing; an upside down Santa Claus in the passenger seat as his traveling companion.

Nancy, Aunt Kate and I spent our last night at Fred's mom's house. In the morning we returned to the "old house" and hooked up the U-Haul. I slowly pulled out of the yard, looking back at the house Fred and I had meticulously restored and decorated. The 150 feet of split rail fence I had put in myself. The small swimming pool we had built for Nancy and her friends to play in. The friendship garden and vegetable gardens Fred and I planted each spring. The large brick patio and barbecue Fred had built and where we had enjoyed many parties with our family, friends and neighbors on warm summer weekends. So much love and so many good memories.

"I'll miss it, won't you?" Nancy craned her neck around.

I nodded. There were too many feelings for me to put into words. My heart physically began to ache. Once again I began to have second thoughts. The same question kept running through my mind. Were we doing the right thing?

We drove up the street to say goodbye to my mother. She walked out to the end of her driveway, tears in her eyes. Seeing her crying nearly broke my heart. We made our promises to each other to call and write every week. As we drove away I watched her in my rear view mirror standing there, looking sadly after us. I turned right onto Coney Street and lost sight of her, but she remained in my heart.

CHAPTER NINETEEN

Living the Florida Dream

We headed down Route # 1. Aunt Kate rode in the front seat with me and Nancy sat in the back seat wedged among boxes, her pet parakeet by her side. My mind swirled between all that I was leaving behind, my family, friends, memories, and all that I was moving toward, a new life, new friends, new memories. My emotions swirled as well. One moment I was gripped with fear, the next I could hardly contain my excitement.

On our first stop for gas, the attendant asked me, "You're going to drive that all the way to Miami yourself?"

A little taken aback, I replied, "Yes."

"Better keep checking the trailer hitch and make sure it's secure. Just jump up and down on it."

As we pulled away from the pump I heard him call after us, "Be careful! And good luck!"

That first night I found out I could not back up the car with the trailer attached. Nancy burst into laughter as I tried, but each time I put the car in reverse the trailer would go in the opposite direction from what I intended. I finally conceded this was one skill I could not master and resigned myself to finding motels I could easily pull in and out of. And I did remember the gas station attendant's suggestion of checking the trailer hitch each morning before we started out.

Two days into the trip we hit rain and heavy traffic. Route # 1 was still a two-lane highway, cars passing each other, whipping in and out of traffic. I gripped the steering wheel tight as one car pulled out from behind us, sped by a long line of cars and trucks ahead of us and barely made it back into his lane before oncoming traffic reached him.

Aunt Kate shook her head in disgust, "He probably won't make it to wherever he is going."

A shiver ran through me as she said it. About an

hour later traffic came to a stop, then slowly inched by a horrible sight. The body of the car that had passed us sat mangled on the side of the road; its upturned engine lay farther away in a field. To upset to go any further we stopped early that night, as did many others.

Fred's and my plan was to meet up in Jacksonville and stay at the home of a couple we knew. When the three of us arrived, we were relieved to see Fred's van sitting in their driveway. We sat down for a delicious home cooked dinner that night and told our stories, so glad to be safe and with our friends.

Fred left early the next morning and we followed close behind, our journey almost over. Arriving in Miami we stayed with Dick and Bette for several days until we had made our final inspection of the house and set up the closing date. What a wonderful sight it was to see the house finished, painted and landscaped. We had been concerned about not being there to watch over the construction, asking for things to righted if they appeared to be going in the wrong direction, but we found nothing amiss.

Leaving the signing with keys in our hands, we headed for our new home, a beautiful three bedroom, two bath ranch with a big back yard. Fred started unpacking the black van and I directed him as to where each piece of furniture would be placed.

Nancy asked if she could stay outside in the front yard under a newly planted ficus tree. I didn't object, thinking it was probably easier to have her out from under foot as Fred carried in furniture and heavy boxes. I watched from my new kitchen window as a young girl, about Nancy's age, crossed the street and ran around the tree talking to Nancy.

"Hiya kid! I'm Stephanie. My house is the yellow one across the street. I'm from Ohio. I'm eight and I live with my aunt and uncle and my dog's name is Abner. Will you be my friend?"

I smiled as I heard Nancy say, "Sure!"

Both girls soon burst through the front door, their hands clasped together.

"Mom! Dad! This is Stephanie! She's my new best friend!"

There stood Stephanie with a big smile on her face, a little imp that we would soon come to love as our own daughter. The girls sat out on the back patio that afternoon and began a friendship that has never ended.

Every day hundreds of people pulled up roots and moved away. They left a town they'd called home for years, a place where they'd grown up, married and settled down. They closed the door behind them on an empty house. Pulling up roots suddenly was not an easy thing. The roots ran deep, the friendships dear, the habits instilled.

In leaving New England, we left behind everything we had known and loved. We left a part of our heritage, the quiet, good kind of life we knew. We left our close knit families, where discipline was the watch word. We left behind the "old house" with its musty smell from the dirt cellar, creaking wood floors and steep stairs leading up to two tiny bedrooms. We left behind Nancy's first steps, her first words, her first day at school, chickenpox, mumps, her falling on the pile of bricks, our romps through the fields in search of blueberries and wild grapes.

In Florida we found a new kind of life. Suburban, where house lots were as small as postage stamps and neighbors were friendly. North Miami was a quite, safe place to live in 1957, filled with palm trees, hibiscus, gardenias and night-flowering jasmine. We loved driving downtown, walking along Bayfront Park, scouring the Miami Public library for books to read, then driving up Biscayne Boulevard and A1A, past miles of wide open stretches of beach.

Nancy started fifth grade in her new school, Norland Elementary, quickly making new friends. Although they were a year apart, she and Steph walked to and from school together each day and in the afternoons rode their bikes around the neighborhood, exploring.

Steph began spending as much time at our home as her own. Most evenings Steph ate dinner at our house, afterward the girls helped each other with their homework. Many evenings it was difficult to separate them and I'd have to issue my, "Girls, it's time to call it a day."

Stephanie would bow her head and pick up her

things. "Bye Mrs. Webster. See you tomorrow, Nan." Then she silently walked across the street toward home.

On weekends there was the inevitable "sleep-over" either at our house or Steph's. She and Nan became inseparable, even going so far as to prick their fingers to become "blood sisters."

We began replacing our memories of New England with those of our new life in Florida, meeting and making new friends along the way. Stephanie's aunt and uncle, Maud and Don, joined us on Saturday evenings for my traditional Boston baked beans and brown bread dinners. We spent most Sunday afternoons with Dick, Bette and Marilyn, the two cousins becoming close friends.

Maud and I soon began our coffee klatches back and forth, sharing our girl's problems. Whenever Nan and Steph had a disagreement, we backed off. Our friendship became too valuable to let the girls' quarrels put space between us. Maud was genuine, taking every step of her life with a bit of wisdom sprinkled with humor. With Maud there was no pretense, no stuffiness, only a gift for loving people.

Our next door neighbors, the Maynards, introduced us to another couple, Mac and Bill. Mac worked as a nurse for a well respected OB/GYN. Trusting her opinion of the doctor she worked for, I made an appointment and took Nancy in for her yearly checkup and last polio vaccine. Finally gone were my fears of her having the inoculations. Dr. Cantor found Nancy to be completely healthy and developing normally.

The one thing Dr. Cantor did suggest was an eye doctor for Nancy. He gave me the name of a doctor he recommended and I called for an appointment. We were surprised and thrilled to find out that Nancy would no longer need to wear glasses. Instead, for the next year, she would use special drops that would correct her weak eye. I thought how easily the first of her crookeds was completely corrected.

1958 was a busy year. In early spring, Fred bought a fourteen foot Chris Craft. I tried to put aside my frugal New England habits. Who could live in Florida without a boat? Nancy loved to sit atop the bow as Fred piloted it out through Haulover Cut, facing forward to catch the spray. We enjoyed our Sundays meandering up the inter-coastal waterway, finding quiet spots to anchor and enjoy our picnic lunch. Nancy took to the water like a porpoise, learning to swim, diving in and under the water, up for a breath of air, then down under again.

One Saturday Fred took Nancy out off Ft. Lauderdale on a father-daughter fishing trip, but instead of catching any fish she ended up throwing up after eating a whole box of Oreo cookies. Too many cookies and a rocking boat did not mix.

We still had to prod Nancy to eat all her vegetables and milk remained her mainstay. After school, with their tall glasses of milk and a plate of cookies, she and Steph would sit on the back patio, poring over books and magazines, working on their scrapbooks. I kept wishing for a few more pounds of flesh on her bones, or at least for her body to stop shooting up so fast.

That summer we made our first trip to Sanibel Island, suggested by one of the couples Fred and I had met in our Bonco group. We fell in love with the island, with its simplicity, peace and quiet. At that time, the only way to reach the island was by ferry from Punta Rassa. What fun we had standing at the front of the ferry as it swished its way through the bay, pelicans flying low over the water beside us. We spent a long weekend walking the beach looking for shells, soon learning the Sanibel Stoop. We were hooked on shelling and came back with bags full of beautiful shells to sift through.

Nancy turned eleven that summer, and I knew that soon the teenage years would begin. I only hoped she would not rush herself in to growing up too fast, and I reminded myself not to push her into things she was not yet ready for. She and Steph began holing themselves up in her bedroom, talking girl talk. Once in a while I had the privilege of being drawn into their discussions.

One day a new girl to our home asked point blank, “Why don’t you let Nan wear lipstick?”

Barely eleven herself, she was adding another layer of red to her already painted lips. Steph sat on Nan’s bed, giggling.

"Aren't you ever going to let her?" the child asked again.

"Someday," I answered.

"But when?" She gave the quiz a third try and added, "What about dates? When can she go out on a date?"

Nan stepped back and began rearranging her horse statues on the top of her shelves. I wondered if she was afraid I'd embarrass her with a "square" answer of mount my "soap box."

"When she's ready," I finally answered.

The young girl shrugged her shoulders and screwed up her lips. I chose not to lecture on the pitfalls of trying to grow up too soon. I sensed she wouldn't be responsive. Maybe, in time. But the time never came. A few weeks later we learned that her family had moved away, apparently in the middle of the night.

In the fall, Fred traded in the Chris Craft for 22-foot prowler, an older boat with a small cabin, head and inboard motor, proudly naming her "Nancy Ann." He found a small marina in Dania and rented dock space. With a larger boat we had more room to take out friends on the weekends, always including Steph. The girls loved to sit on the back end of the boat, singing to their hearts content.

One weekend Fred went up to check on the boat and found it partially submerged. Heartsick, he arranged to have the boat raised and trailered home, where it sat for over a year, until he finished refurbishing it from the inside out.

To take his mind off the boat and the work that lay ahead of him, we started taking weekend drives. One Sunday we found a little town just north of us called Davie, a horse town, famous for its yearly rodeo and acres of orange groves. We started spending our Sundays driving past field after field of cows and horses, stopping at Flamingo Groves to pick up our fresh oranges for the coming week. Most Sundays Stephanie came with us, the girls sitting in the back seat counting horses, whispering and giggling.

We started dreaming of perhaps owning a piece of land there someday, of designing our own home and building it ourselves. At times I thought back to the weekend trips to Vermont Fred and I had made in the months before our marriage, trying to find a farm to buy. Perhaps our dream would finally come true.

CHAPTER TWENTY

Learning to Ride

It was inevitable for the issue of horses to come up again. At first, Nancy was content to count how many horses she saw each Sunday on our drives through Davie. Fred made it a point to stop by the side of the road to let her and Steph pet some horses, feed them carrots and talk to them. Her horse figurine collection grew so large Fred built extra shelves above her desk.

Pony rides came next, but they were only a teaser. She soon grew too tall for the ponies and began pestering us for riding lessons.

"Mom, there's a riding stable near Greynold's Park," Nancy said to me one day when she came in from school. "Do you think... Mom? Did you hear me?" She nudged my arm.

"Yes, honey. I was just thinking." I hugged her shoulder.

"Do you think daddy will let me take lessons?" She leaned her head on my arm.

"The only way to find out is to ask him."

"Okay, I will when he gets home." She turned to go down the hall.

"After supper," I called out. "Wait 'till after supper."

"Okay, mom. Okay."

Fathers have a soft spot for daughters, especially if they are an only child. Fred was no exception. Nancy was his world, as she was mine. He could not refuse her request.

The stables she had mentioned had many horses. Spirited, well trained horses for the more experienced rider, all the way to the gentle old mares for the beginners. Nancy started in the beginners' class with Tom. Tanned, weathered Tom, who had seen many years in the saddle and knew the importance of basic instruction.

Nancy was excited that first day as she climbed the

steps of the mounting block. Tom held the reins of a brown mare and brought her forward.

"Come on now. Up you go." He motioned. "There. No, your left foot. Put your left foot in the stirrup. Hold the reins in your left hand, grab the saddle and pull yourself up and over."

She sat proud and straight in the saddle as Tom adjusted the length of the stirrups. He led her into the ring with the other beginners.

"Toes up. Heels down." He called out to each child. "Hold your reins firm, not too tight. Relax those reins and nudge your horse's belly with your heel." He led the first horse around and the others followed. "Straight! Keep those backs straight! And keep your heels down." He tapped the foot of one child. "Always remember, toes up, heels down."

Nancy sat well, but appeared so small on top of such a huge animal. She listened to Tom's every word, trying to remember her hands, feet, knees and back all at once.

"How'd I do?" she asked as she sat between us on the way home.

"Fine," I answered. "Did you like it?"

"Mmm," she said, pulling her knees up to her chest and hugging her jeans, grimy with horse sweat.

"Just remember one thing," Fred said. "Being off guard around a horse or losing control of a spirited one and you are in big trouble."

"Oh, daddy, I promise I won't."

From then on her weekly ride became a routine thing. Tom calling out, hooves kicking up the dirt faster and faster, backs straighter, hands more sure on the reins, knees and heels learning their power to direct and control. Nancy sat well, her slim long legs and feet reaching down into the stirrups, long slim arms and fingers grasping the reins. She would be a good rider, maybe even a great one. Visions of shows and ribbons and cheers, parental pride working overtime. Just so long as it stayed in our heads, no harm. We smiled at our child and welled up inside.

Each time around the ring, Nancy turned to look at us with her smile of elation, pure joy, like nothing I'd ever seen before. Riding truly meant that much to her. There had to be new clothes, Jodhpurs, shirts, leather boots, not only for looks, but also for safety in the saddle. Several weeks later, Nancy was unusually excited and impatient as we drove the six miles to the stables.

"I get to canter today."

"Oh," I said, pulling the bow tighter on one of her pigtails.

"Uhuh. Tom says I'm ready."

Later in the ring, her horse kicked up the dirt faster and faster as she directed the mare from a walk into a trot. At Tom's instruction, she moved into a canter, a little jumpy at first, until she got the feeling of the gait. Soon her body, arms and legs were rising and lowering in rhythmic ease, her face flushed. She threw a quick smile our way, then down at her horse. At Tom's command she brought her horse to a halt, then walked on, occasionally leaning forward, stroking the horse's mane. For this hour the mare was her horse. When class was over she dismounted, slipped off the bridle and reins, replacing them with a halter and lead line.

"Gotta walk her to cool her down." She touched the horse's moist neck. Back and forth she strolled, the mare obediently following. Often she would let the mare catch up to her so she could turn and pat her nose.

By March of 1959 Nancy had grown several more inches and now reached my chin. She was still lean, but healthy. I marveled at the litheness of her body and her boundless energy. Her body seemed to be growing straight. I guess, unless the thought was placed before me, I didn't think about abnormalities. Her legs were long and slim, just like her dad's. I kept thinking she would catch up in weight when she stopped growing in height. At eleven, she still had a long way to go.

During that summer, Fred was laid off from his carpentry work. We tightened our belts, hoping he would find work soon. After several weeks of making the rounds in Miami with no luck, he answered an ad placed by a company looking for experienced carpenters to work in Nassau, building homes in Lyford Cay. Fred applied for the job and was immediately hired. The company paid for his flight to Nassau and put him up in a company home located on the ocean, complete with a maid named Pearl to cook and clean for him.

At first his letters to me sounded as if he were living in a dream world; working during the day, swimming in the ocean each evening, enjoying weekend fishing trips. As the weeks progressed his letters reflected his growing disenchantment. He was homesick for Nancy and me, even missed my home cooking.

One day I received a letter from him saying:

Arlene,

I'm finishing the job here and will be home before long.

Love,
Fred

I literally dropped everything and radioed a message back:

Arriving on the next flight. Please meet us.
Arlene

I thought if Nancy and I could be there with him, he might change his mind.

When we boarded the plane in Miami, Nancy was bursting with excitement. She would be spending her twelfth birthday in the islands. After seating ourselves, the stewardess approached.

"Cocktails?"

"Mmm, yes, I think so."

"And what would you like?" She looked over at Nancy.

"Tomato juice?" Nancy was quite taken with the luxury and service, the anticipation of the days before us.

We spent the next several weeks, indeed, living in a dream world. We stayed in an old English house with a sea grape and palm tree lined path leading to a private beach. Pearl came each day to prepare and serve our meals. She washed and cleaned, singing as she worked. She picked and set red hibiscus blossoms in small containers all around the house.

Each morning after Fred left for work, Nancy and I took the winding path to the beach, chameleons criss-crossing in front of us. We swam in the calm, clear water, walked the quiet beach. We swam again in the evenings with Fred. He taught Nancy how to snorkel and the two of them loved to float on the gentle waves and watch the stingrays glide gracefully below them.

We enjoyed our trips to "town" visiting the straw market, viewing the replicas of the British crown jewels, and climbing up the Queen's staircase. The wife of one of the developers graciously invited Nancy and I over for lunch one day and then took us for a drive around Lyford Cay. We stopped on a high hill overlooking the sea, then walked down to a cave hole where we knelt to watch the sea come in and dash against the rocks way below us.

With no housework or cooking to do, I relished my treasured free time to spend on several writing projects. Despite our being there, Fred grew more and more disheartened with the job. Sadly, we packed our suitcases and headed back to Miami in time for Nancy to start seventh grade.

Starting junior high, Nancy left Steph, who was a year younger, behind. She missed Steph, but the girls continued to play every day after school, remaining as close as ever. In one of her new classes Nancy met Jill, a very lively, petite, outgoing young girl. They quickly became close friends and remained so all throughout the rest of school. Jill shared a love of horses with Nan, both girls often riding together. Both girls fell in love with and cried over a racehorse named Carry Back.

Nancy continued her riding lessons, graduating from Tom to Lester, who would continue her training, advancing her to more difficult horses.

One Sunday we took our usual afternoon drive up to Davie. We passed ranch after ranch, some advertising riding. Nancy begged the inevitable question.

"Can I daddy?"

Why not? She'd had a good lesson the day before, she knew how to sit, give signals and she had advanced to cantering. If the horse was well trained, why not let her have an extra ride this weekend?

We stopped at one of the ranches and inquired. With no one there except the owner, the horse and us, Nancy mounted, and settled into the western saddle. She kicked the black belly. The horse took a few steps and halted. She kicked again. He turned and came back to us.

"You're sure he's okay for her?" I asked.

"Yes, ma'am." He adjusted the stirrups, turned the horse around, heading him in the direction of the open field.

An uneasy felling hit me, a split second urge to have her dismount. But before I could open my mouth, the man laid his whip on the horse's flank. The horse took off at a full gallop as he headed for the open field. Was she ready? Could she stay with him?

As the horse raced forward, Nancy held tight to the reins, hugging his belly with her knees, her toes pointed up in the stirrups. She leaned forward slightly and kept her seat, her hair flying in the wind.

My pride and fear were mixed. Suddenly, without warning, the black devil stopped short, making a quarter turn to the right. Nancy flew up in the air. Up, up, up, then down, out of sight behind the fence.

"My God, he threw her!" I cried as the horse galloped back to us, saddle empty, stirrups swinging free.

All three of us raced across the field, around the fence and to the spot where Nancy lay, her head almost buried in the black dirt. There was dirt in her hair, dirt in her mouth, dirt in her nose and her eyes were closed. She had blacked out.

Fred reached her first, knelt and gathered her in his arms, tapping her face. He began to wipe the dirt from her nose so she could breathe. Dropping to my knees, I reached over. Fred, knowing my panic, held me back. Nancy's eyes opened, rolled around and closed. Fred tapped her again.

"Nancy, Nancy. You're all right. Open your eyes." His voice was calm and soothing.

Nancy's eyelids fluttered and opened. Tears mixed with the black dirt as she began sobbing uncontrollably. "Daddy! Mommy!"

Fred stood up with Nancy in his arms and carried her back to the ranch house. We bathed her bruises and helped her stand up.

"I'm okay," she insisted.

"Are you sure? Your legs, your arms, your back,

they don't hurt anywhere?

"No, mom. I'm okay. I want to go home."

We drove in silence, Nancy leaning against my arm. Thank God for the black dirt. It had been a cushion for her fall. Thank God for Tom and Lester's instructions. Toes up, heels down. She had been thrown free instead of being dragged.

Fred had been right. Horses could be killers. Should we insist she stop riding? I looked down at my rumpled little girl in her dirty blue jeans, her eyes closed against the round of my shoulder. I knew the answer. We couldn't. No more than we could stop her from growing up and away from us some day. She would have to learn to outwit whatever horse she rode. That was the only answer.

Nancy appeared to have no ill effects from her fall. The next week on the way to the stables, I wondered about her emotional reaction. Fear was easily planted and if not faced squarely, could become imbedded.

As we walked toward the horse stalls and the mounting block, Nancy skipped ahead. "I get to ride Red today." She turned back to me for a second, grinned, then hurried up the steps. When Red was led over to her, she reached for the reins, swung herself up into the saddle, then turned her horse at a slow walk into the intermediate ring.

Lester stood in the center, crop in hand. He signaled for a slow trot. Nancy moved Red forward, falling easily into the rhythm of posting. Round and round. Lester watched each child, turning occasionally to spot any riding fault he might have missed.

"Okay! Halt!" he shouted.

Nancy brought Red to a complete stop not far from where I stood at the rail. She sat still, holding Red at attention as Lester walked from one youngster to another, checking toes, heels, knees, hands and backs. Stepping back to the center again, he placed his left hand on his hips.

"Put your horses into a fast canter for three rounds, then into a gallop. Watch your backs and hands." He cracked his whip to the ground.

Nancy leaned forward for a moment. Was she afraid? A moment later she straightened, urging Red into a smooth canter. Around she rode, once, twice, three times. Then she pulled Red up short and leaned forward again.

I watched and waited, the moment dragging. She patted Red's sleek neck and mouthed words I could not hear. Suddenly Red took off in a gallop. On the first turn, I leaned over the rail, relieved. Lester cracked his whip into the ground again, each horse galloping faster. Soon Nancy's legs and knees were soaked in sweat from Red's warm flanks. I stood back. This was her little victory.

After her lesson, Nancy cooled Red down, then worked with the currycomb and brush. She brushed and smoothed, patted and talked, then put Red back in his stall.

"Okay, mom. I'm ready to go home now."

TWENTY ONE

Something is Happening

In the spring of 1960, Fred and I realized part of our long held dream. We bought a piece of land in Davie, a beautiful acre with a thick grove of melaleuka trees. We walked the property each Sunday, trying to decide where we would eventually build our new home. Mom and pop, having enjoyed spending the past three winters with us, decided on buying the acre next to us to build a small winter home for themselves.

That summer Nancy and I spent our first full week on Sanibel. The old ferry carried us from Punta Rassa across the three miles of San Carlos Bay. After docking, I drove over the huge wooden planks onto the dirt road leading by the old post office. To the left curved a narrow cart path leading to the almost deserted lighthouse. To the right, the dirt road curved its way onto Periwinkle Way, past the Sea Horse Shop, where we stopped to browse and I purchased my first copy of Anne Morrow Lindbergh's *Gift from the Sea*. We shopped for groceries at old Bailey's General Store, continued on down Periwinkle Way, driving under the canopy of Australian pines, then on to the small apartment on the beach I had rented for the week.

We enjoyed the instant camaraderie of the other beachcombers, collecting conchs and welks, olive shells and jewel boxes, sand dollars and coquina. We checked our tide charts daily for low tide, the best time for shelling. Often we plodded through the muck on the bay side near Bailey's General Store, digging for Kings Crowns.

We walked the beach and sat in the shade of palm and pine trees, with nothing to mar the peace. The tumble of the surf on shore and the occasional call of a lone bird were the only sounds to break the silence.

We loved dining on our own balcony, watching the ever changing sea, watching as the sun set and evening closed in, the water off shore becoming a sea of phosphorescence riding in on each wave. There was that *something* about a place where you hold hands with nature, a perfect place for mother and daughter to draw close.

Nancy also enjoyed summer school at the stables. She attended for two weeks, was given her "own" horse to take care of, feed, groom, and ride every day. She always started the day starched, fresh and clean, coming home smudgy, sweaty and smelling of the stables, but in complete happiness.

She knew she had to ride frequently to be ready for horse shows. Not the professional ones held at Dinner Key Auditorium each year, but special shows held at the stables. In her first show we watched Nancy mount Red, then sit ready and anxious to start. She leaned over to pat and talk secret communicative words to her horse. When her class was called, she entered the ring smiling, her back straight, her knees firm, her hands steady. She followed the orders - trotting, fast canters, figure eights, mounting and dismounting. When the judging was complete she stood in line with all the other hopeful youngsters gazing at their parents, all wishing for the blue ribbon.

When the judges announced, *"The blue ribbon goes to Nancy Webster,"* her eyes opened wide. She walked Red in perfect form to the judges where she was presented with her first blue ribbon. All the way home her fingers kept running over the satiny surface of the blue ribbon, her eyes half closed in elation.

We knew then, it was not just a passing fancy, a momentary whim. After her riding, she was willing to spend fifteen to twenty minutes walking a horse to cool him off, then brush, groom, pick hooves, clean out stalls, all the things necessary to properly take care of a horse. Her love for horses was one of the purest kinds of love, the kind of love where there was communication between the animal and her, a love that could not easily be extinguished.

Dentist appointments filled our calendar the rest of that year. After her cleaning and fillings were completed, our dentist recommended Nancy see an orthodontist for her crooked teeth. He gave me the names of several and after visiting each, Nancy chose the one she felt most comfortable with. Thus started her ordeal with appointments, x-rays, impressions, braces and rubber bands. She tried to be good-natured about the process, but at times frustration took over. There were favorite foods she could not eat, especially popcorn, and no matter how careful she was her rubber bands kept breaking. She dreaded each year when the metal bands were removed and she went in for teeth cleaning and to be checked for cavities. Then the whole process started again with new impressions, more metal and rubber bands. Three years after her first appointment, her orthodontist was satisfied with the results and Nancy was fitted for her retainer. Finally, the second of her crookeds was taken care of.

We still had no inkling of the third.

How quickly the years passed. Most of all I remember how normal everything seemed. Certainly not perfect, but just so normal. How happy and secure we were that we had make our decision to move to Florida. Fred enjoyed his work and increasing responsibilities of construction superintendent on several large projects. Nancy, Steph and Jill were the happy girlfriend threesome, including Marilyn whenever they could. Mom and pop continued to enjoy their winters with us. We had our ups and downs, but there were no more thoughts of measles, mumps, or polio. We were blessed nothing tragic had touched our lives. We stood protectively over Nancy, guiding her spiritually and physically into the ways of all round health. She responded, proving a credit to us in church, school, at home.

How little did I know how much things were about to change. As I look back I saw an inkling of changes that the summer Nancy turned fourteen. As we neared Sanibel Island for our mother-daughter week together, Nancy began noticing the clumps of sea oats hugging the sand dunes, and the posted signs:

"UNLAWFUL TO PICK SEA OATS."

"Mmm. Pretty," she said. "Wish we could pick some. But I guess we shouldn't."

"Uhuh," came my automatic reply.

A few minutes of driving in silence ended suddenly. "Mom! Stop right here!"

I looked over at Nancy, then pulled alongside the road and turned off the ignition. Between us and the sea were rolling sand dunes topped with sea oats.

"Let's pick some mom. If we hurry, no one will see us."

I hesitated. No answer came. Yet, here, looking out at the natural beauty, something touched me.

"We'll go see," I said.

We both got out of the car and walked between the dunes toward the beach. On the way we could see where dune buggy tires had made tracks in the sand. Some of the sea oat clumps were crushed, the golden stalks lying on the sand, their leaf filled limbs no longer swaying in the breeze. Doomed.

"Here, we can have these," I said. So with a paring knife from my picnic basket, I easily cut off the flattened sea oats. Back in the car I set them down on the seat between us. Nice. At least we can enjoy them, I thought.

I started the car up slowly, but stopped abruptly alongside the next dune. There, staked out on the top was a large sign:

"CONDOMINIUMS TO BE ERECTED ON THIS SITE. COMPLETION BY..."

My eyes blurred. I dabbed them with a tissue. Must be my hay fever. My thoughts were fragmented words - earth, man, nourishment, sea oats, sand dunes, the beach, preservation, a higher plan, harmony, survival.

Nancy broke my philosophical babblings. "Didn't you see the sign way back?"

I shook my head.

"You know," she continued. "Grown-ups say one thing and do another. Sometimes you don't make any sense at all."

By the time she was fifteen, Nancy had mastered roller-skating, bicycling, and horsemanship. In the water she could match any mermaid. We were, I admit, a bit proud of our offspring.

Before we knew it, it was 1962 and Nancy started 10th grade. Her high school years had begun. But to our surprise she seemed to change overnight from smiling and happy to quiet and withdrawn. She kept up with her schoolwork, continuing to make good grades, but she was not at social as we might have hoped for. The boys didn't call very often. She didn't want to go to parties or dances at school. She did keep up with her Sunday school classes, meeting and becoming friends with Pam, and joined a young women's group offering weekly meetings, which she sporadically attended.

Horses became the center of her life, almost to the exclusion of everything else. Nancy continued with her riding lessons, advancing through several other horses and then was given Miss Arlene, one of the top horses in the stable. With Miss Arlene Nancy went on to win several more ribbons in school shows, advanced into dressage classes and finally jumping classes. Riding two nights a week and on Saturdays, along with equitation classes and summer horse camp, seemed, at least for a while, to stem the longing for her own horse. One of the drawbacks of learning to ride was learning to fall and Nancy had her share of spills. But each time she would stand up, dust herself off and remount her horse. Courage and persistence, traits she would need all too soon in her life.

I lost my father in the fall of 1963. When word came, Fred was at work, Nan was at school. As the shock and numbness set in the only thing I could think of was rushing across the street to Maud's kitchen. She would know how I felt.

"It hurts like hell," she said. "So, cry it out."

I did. She made coffee and we sat, talking. Later, on our way to the airport, she assured me she'd look after my family. Her parting words to me were, "It may be hard to believe now, but in time the pain will be gone and you'll feel only the sweetness of the good memories."

I left Nancy in Fred's care to travel home to say my good-byes. My father had been a quiet man. A thinking man who rarely showed outward affection. How did I know he even cared? I had had to be receptive to his cues. The beam in his eyes whenever I made the honor roll in school, his interest in my music lessons by suffering through the torture of listening to a beginning violinist. And his pride when I finally mastered "La Paloma," asking me to play it for hours on end. It was his way of saying, "I love you."

Crushed by the loss, I tried to remember back to papa and his woodworking shop. Papa with his head in a book or sitting at the kitchen table doodling cartoons. Mutt and Jeff were his best. How papa loved listening to good music. He thought Glenn Miller and Benny Goodman were the desecration of the memory of Mozart and Schubert and the ruining of the younger generation. How much he and mama had enjoyed spending the past several winters with us, how much he had enjoyed sitting out in our back yard, soaking up the Florida sun.

"Yes, papa. I remember. I remember so well, all the good things."

For several years Nancy had not had her usual checkups with Dr. Cantor. I didn't persist, as she had no illness or problems that required attention. Our time had been spent on eye doctor, dentist and orthodontist appointments. I wonder now, if I had taken her each year to see Dr. Cantor for her exams, would he have detected the scoliosis earlier? Would it have prevented her from major surgery? In the 60's there was no mandatory testing for scoliosis.

Nancy had just turned sixteen when I began noticing the hitch to her right side. One morning as she started down our front walk on her way to school, I called out after her, "For heavens sake, walk straight!"

"Okay, mom. Okay!" she called back.

I went about my housework that day, thinking nothing more about it. Teenagers had a way of slouching, twisting and bending into numerous contortions anyway. Pliable, lithe, they stayed still scarcely for a moment. Nancy was no exception.

Each morning after, I noticed the same hitching position. "My goodness, will you straighten up?"

"I am. I am."

"No, you're not."

"I can't straighten any more, mom."

What was there about a hint of realization? When that realization concerns things you don't want to face, you shut it out. I kept telling myself it was simply her posture.

She was growing so fast, so tall and lean. Perhaps that too was why at times she appeared more tired than usual and would plunk herself down on her bed or on the couch to study instead of sitting up. She mentioned a tired feeling in her back. I thought perhaps she had just overdone. Kids did get periods of exhaustion. Besides with all the things she was doing, horseback riding, swimming, skin diving, biking...

Clothes became one of our major battlegrounds. She was unhappy with everything she wore. Having sewn all my life, I tried to make the latest styles for her, but nothing seemed to fit right. She'd stand in front of her mirror, turn around, pull and tug, and maybe make two or three changes before she was satisfied. Even store bought clothes hung unevenly. It never occurred to me to check her back.

Sophistication also had set in and with it a tight lid on privacy. She no longer dashed from the bathroom to her bedroom wrapped in only a towel. If her bedroom door was closed, I usually knocked before entering. Once, though, I did open her door without knocking and found her turning around in front of her mirror, a concerned look on her face.

"For Pete sakes, mom! I'm dressing!" She grabbed for her robe.

I left quickly, forgetting what prompted my intrusion in the first place. However, I couldn't ignore the fact. Something was happening.

In her junior year Nancy tried desperately to get out of having to take physical education. There was no way to excuse her with no physical impairment that we knew of. She finally admitted to how much she hated having to take showers after gym class, embarrassed to have to strip in front of the other girls, trying to cover up with what barely could be considered a towel.

That same year, Lester gave Nancy the top horse in the stables. Tammy became her greatest challenge. Many nights she would come home, frustrated. "Mom, why can't I ride Tammy? I just can't get the feeling for her." She had not yet been able to reach that connection when horse and rider become one. Lester kept urging her to think out the solution, but the more she tried, the more frustrated she became.

One evening Nancy lay on the sectional in our living room. "Look, mom, my right leg is longer than my left."

"Come on now. Don't be silly," I said.

"I'm not. Honest." She turned to her dad. "You look dad."

We both looked. One foot did seem to extend beyond the other.

"You're just doing that. You're stretching your right leg."

"No, I'm not, mom."

"All right. Stand up."

She did. For the first time in months Nancy stood still and let us really look at her. Her shorts made it easy to compare on leg with the other. Her right hip did appear higher than her left. In fact, when I felt her left side, she seemed to have no hip at all.

From that moment on, we realized something was wrong.

TWENTY TWO

Senior Year

In September 1964, Nancy started her senior year of high school. She and Stephanie were still close, but Steph had begun moving in a different direction from Nancy, dating one of the most popular boys in school. Steph tried to include Nancy in on things, but Nancy continued to shy away from boys and parties. The same held true with Jill. The girls remained close, sharing several classes, but Jill began spending more time with the young man she was dating, limiting her time with Nancy.

Nancy had signed up for her second year of art class. There she was reunited with Pam, who had spent most of the past year homebound, recovering from Harrington Rod surgery. With Pam, Nancy opened up and began to talk about the hitch in her clothes; her thoughts that one leg was longer than the other. Pam kept encouraging her to see her doctor, Dr. Robert Keiser. Each time Pam came over she talked to Fred and I about how her surgery to straighten her spine had changed her life.

But our Nancy? Crooked? Of course not. She couldn't be. She was perfect. Had been perfect. Was perfect now. But, much as I tried, I couldn't push the thought away anymore. Poor Pam. I remembered Nancy visiting her in the hospital and at home as she had lain in her cast. Nancy like that? No. I wouldn't think of it. Then, when I did finally mention my fears, friends, trying to reassure, would say, "Oh she's all right. She doesn't look bad. Besides, it's best to leave the spine alone."

"Mom," Nancy said one day, "Why don't you go see Pam's folks. They can tell you all about it."

I didn't want to go and pry. I didn't know them. I hardly knew Pam, except for the times she had come to our house to talk about her surgery. I didn't want to go, more because it would be an outright admission. After that, there would have to be acceptance. I wasn't ready to accept what I think I already knew.

We finally did visit Pam's parents. They talked. We listened in rigid silence. When we got home, I called and made an appointment with Dr. Cantor.

"Look here," he said. He asked Nancy to bend forward on the examining table. He traced the line of her spine. I saw a definite curve and a bulging in her left shoulder area. After her exam, Dr. Cantor met with us in his office. He talked to us reassuringly and gave us the name of an orthopedic diagnostician, Dr. Baird, in Hialeah.

I called Dr. Baird's office and scheduled an appointment for early October. After his exam and x-rays he sat and talked with us, giving us his findings and opinion. He was trying to be warm and kind, but his words hit me cold. I sat transfixed before Nancy's x-ray. I looked at what appeared to be a reversed S shape. Then I listened.

"Your daughter has a severe spinal curvature," he said. "She definitely needs surgery. It is a long procedure, three years or more and once started, there is no turning back."

"The cost?" I barely whispered.

"In the thousands. No more than a fine new car."

Nancy asked the inevitable question, "Would I be able to horseback ride afterward?"

"I wouldn't advise it," he answered.

It was all too much. Too much to absorb all at once. We drove home in silence, the doctor's written summation sitting in my lap.

<u>MEDICAL HISTORY</u>

This 17 year old girl (17 on July 20) is noted to have a curve of the spine approximately a year or so ago. Asymptotic.

<u>Physical Examination</u>

Exam shows a moderately severe left lumbar, right dorsal scoliosis with deformity of the thoracic cage. Moderate flexibility of the lumbar curve. The right crest is slightly higher than the left crest.

<u>EXRAY EXAMINATION</u>

Roentgenograms show a moderately severe curve on

the wet films estimated approximately 60 to 70 degrees.

TREATMENT

Recommend probable surgical correction.

Duke B. Baird M.D.

There it was in black and white. We could no longer ignore it.

"I won't have it," Nancy told us that evening. "If I can't ever ride again, I just won't have it."

We left it at that. Where would we find the time, anyway? Nancy was caught up in all the activities of her senior year. The holidays were fast approaching, then soon enough there would be her final exams, senior banquet and graduation.

In early January of 1965, Nancy did consent to see Pam's Dr. Keiser. In fact, I sensed a real wanting to. I set up an appointment at the spinal clinic at Variety Children's Hospital. We sat impatiently in a waiting room filled with young, noisy children. Nancy, nearing her eighteenth birthday, fidgeted in her seat, uncomfortable in the midst of all the young patients; no one even close to her age.

After a thorough exam and more x-rays, Dr. Keiser wrote on Nancy's chart. "Scoliosis." There before us were her latest films clearly showing the reversed S where a straight spine should be.

"Surgery is definitely needed," he said as several other doctors, pressing in around him, agreed.

With Nancy beside me, I stood back and closed my eyes tight for a second. Then I opened them and focused on the little dots in the ceiling squares above me. Anytime I didn't want the tears to come, I found a way to stop them.

Nancy and I listened carefully to his every word. Her curves had progressed from last fall, now measuring 50-degrees thoracic and 70-degrees lumbar. The rotation of her spine was putting pressure on both her heart and left lung. In his opinion, she needed surgery. He felt there were no other options.

"The important thing to remember is that we don't put a child through such extensive surgery purely for cosmetic reasons. Without the operation, in time, Nancy will possibly become a semi-invalid with severe pain and arthritis of the spine. Although the process is lengthy, success depends in large part upon the patient's full co-operation. With this surgery Nancy will have the opportunity for a relatively normal life."

"Think about it," he said in his calm, sure voice. Although he did not want to rush us, he impressed upon us the need to make a decision soon. Variety Children's Hospital would not accept Nancy after her eighteenth birthday.

Even though we expected the diagnosis, we both walked out of the clinic in shock. On the drive home neither one of us spoke; each of us closed off into our own thoughts.

I tried as best I could to explain to Fred all that we had been told. We talked late into the night. Make a decision? We just wanted to shove it aside and forget about it. But we knew we couldn't. It stood out before us, a demanding a decision we felt we had no right to make. We could guide and advise, but we couldn't make the final decision.

How could we, her parents, make the right decision? And what was the right decision, anyway? To undergo a major operation with months, perhaps years of recovery? Or, without it, realize the fact her spine would continue to curve and she would have severe pain in later years, possibly to the point of being a semi-invalid?

For the first time we knew we could not think and feel in her place. She had the right to decide her future. And so we took the only way out, we decided to let Nancy make the final decision.

TWENTY THREE

The Decision

At first, Nancy shoved the decision aside too, completely ignoring it. Each time we asked her if she'd made her decision she told us, "I won't have it. Not if I can't ever ride horses again. I just won't!"

I felt as if a wall were rising between us. The best medical authorities had strongly advised the surgery, but we could not pressure her. She had to come to the answer herself. We passed the days and weeks after Dr. Keiser's diagnosis by skirting the subject, avoiding it almost altogether, as if it would go away.

But, we knew it wouldn't. It wouldn't go away any more than the knowledge that her spine was curving more each day. I was conscious of it every waking moment. I watched her walk and bend and stretch. No amount of posture exercises could make her straight. She needed the surgery. Her whole future depended on her having it, but we would not, could not force her. She had to find the answer for herself. What a testing and searching. Her patches of silence between forced frivolities bore this out.

In April a letter came. It was from a well meaning relative, who would never have said or done anything intentionally to hurt us. *"Yes,"* the letter said. *"I noticed the curvature this past summer. I should think you and Nancy would jump at the chance to have the operation. After all, she must think of how she looks. Clothes. Boys. And marriage someday."*

Jump at the chance to undergo major spinal surgery? To be immobile in casts for six months? Take the risks that accompanied such a traumatic experience?

I read the letter again and my anger grew. Clothes? Boys? Marriage? Think of the way she looked? Was that really the important thing? Was that really the reason such an operation should be performed? What if brilliant, dedicated men, like Dr. Harrington and our Dr. Keiser, hadn't advanced the surgery? What if Nancy couldn't have had the operation? Would she have been put on a back shelf in a closet somewhere, unsuitable for life, not worthy, because by some quirk of fate she had become less than perfect? Was a human being's worth contained in the perfection of the body? Shouldn't it rather be what he or she has made of their life with what they have been given?

I read the letter a third time and my anger began to subside. The letter had been written out of love for Nancy, even though the thoughts were a little lopsided.

That afternoon I knelt on hands and knees in the back yard, weeding, completely forgetting I had left the letter open on the kitchen table. Was it some subconscious pull that made me do it? I'll never know.

Near three o'clock, I heard the front door open and close. Nancy shouted out her usual, "Hi, mom!" Then the house was quiet. I assumed she was changing and I continued to pile weeds in a heap. I would soon be done and we could have a coke together.

"Mom?" Nancy suddenly plunked herself down beside me, Indian fashion, on the grass.

I looked up, brushed the black dirt from my work gloves. "I'm just about done now and we can have a snack. Okay?"

"Mom? I've made up my mind."

"Oh? I sat down beside her.

"Yes. I've made up my mind to have the surgery."

I looked up into her eyes, knowing she had made her decision. My mind raced, trying to grasp the right words.

"I saw the letter," she added. "I read it, mom."

"I hadn't meant for you..."

"I know," she cut in. "I'm glad I read it though."

"Those aren't the reasons for making up your mind, are they?"

"No, they aren't, mom. They aren't my reasons. Not my first reasons anyway. I remember what Dr. Keiser said."

"Then?"

"They're my second set of reasons. She's right. You know she is mom. Such things are important. I do want to be like everyone else. I do want a straight back. And, I do want to get married someday."

At that moment I wanted to reach over, hug her tight, try to blot out the words that had prompted her to finally make the decision she would have eventually made in her own way. I knew instinctively when my child was hurt. Still part child, but almost a woman, I couldn't kiss the hurt and make it go away.

Nancy jumped up. "Call Dr. Keiser, will you, mom? Almost forgot, Steph and I are going to the beach tomorrow after school. Gotta go see her now. Okay?"

"Okay," I answered.

Sure. It was okay. Everything would be okay.

I called Dr. Keiser's office early the next morning. A few days later we entered his office. I shall never forget the coolness of the room, yet the warmth of his simple greeting.

"Hello," he said. After shaking our hands, he motioned for us to sit down. I remember the smell of the leather and wood and his dark grained massive desk, across which many a child's records must have passed.

Nancy took the chair in front of him. I took the one to the side. And that was how I felt. Outside, yet close to the turmoil I was sure she still held within her.

She sat as straight as she could with a 50/70 curvature. Her pale blue and white A line dress accented the freshness of her seventeen years. She looked directly at the doctor to whom she would soon be entrusting her whole future.

He leaned forward, his arms resting on the clean glass top the desk. I noticed his hands. Not large. Not small. But hands with a steadiness in their movement. And skill and strength.

"He is one of the best orthopedic surgeons in the south." Those words I had heard more than once. I based my faith on their validity. His dark eyes shone through rimmed glasses. His face, neither young nor old, was one of distinction. He had the air of a doctor, that comforting, knowing air.

"So. You've made up your mind, have you?" He directed his words toward Nancy.

She twitched a little in her chair and sat up

straighter. She answered with a faint, "Yes."

He glanced at me briefly, then looked straight at Nancy again. He repeated words we had heard before, words almost too hard to accept.

"This is a lengthy procedure. You do understand that?"

Nancy nodded and forced a smile.

"Once the surgery is performed, there is no going back. You will have to see it through."

I could hear a door open and close somewhere close by. My mind floated like the air from the air-conditioning vents. Downward. Upward. Around. I touched my cheek and felt almost nothing. I swallowed and my throat was dry. *Lengthy procedure. No going back. Months in casts.* His words came to me as if from space. He outlined the surgery. The insertion of rods. The fusion. The post-operative period. He left nothing unsaid.

We had to be willing to go the whole way. We assured him we were.

"Good. And now, there are just a few things more I want to say before making the arrangements."

His seeming bluntness ended and his manner softened with the same warmth he first had shown us. "The success of the procedure depends on our joint co-operation. I don't think I have to concern myself there."

We shook our heads. He could depend on us. We would not let him down.

He leaned back a little in his chair. "There is one last point I want to make again. We do not perform such major surgery purely for cosmetic reasons. Our main concern is the patient's ability to lead a normal life. This, and only this, justifies putting you through such a long procedure. It is important you both realize what I am saying.

Nancy and I both nodded.

"Nancy?"

"Yes, sir?" She leaned forward in her chair.

"Just what is your reason for wanting the surgery?"

Nancy grasped the arms of the chair firmly, raised her head high and answered, "I just want a straight back."

Simple. Direct. Honest. She had summed it up.

He smiled, then called for his secretary. With our

agreement, he set the date for surgery. July ninth. Nancy would be admitted into the hospital on July seventh, thirteen days before her eighteenth birthday.

We were about done with all the necessary details. We could go now, I thought. Nancy stood up and approached the desk. "May I ask something?"

"Of course, you may," Dr. Keiser smiled up at Nancy.

She began slowly. "Dr. Keiser, when the operation is over, and later, much later, like a year or two, when I'm out of the cast and all," she hesitated, swallowed and continued, "Can I ride horses again?"

Dr. Keiser leaned further back in his chair. I heard it squeak in the silence of the room. His face took on a seriousness and he folded his arms.

I felt a pain jab right through the middle of my chest. Why did she have to ask? Dr. Baird had told her she would never ride again. Why bring all the hurt back? I closed my eyes, trying to shut out the question.

When I opened them, I saw a smile on Dr. Keiser's face. "If everything goes as planned, and after a reasonable length of time, you can go back to all normal activity."

"You mean I can ride?"

In his professional manner, he repeated, "You can go back to all normal activity."

Nancy's hands flew to her mouth. Perhaps she was holding back a YIPPEE! Or a squeal. Neither she nor I could find any other words except, "Thank you, doctor!"

We shook his hand, turned and left his office, fairly gliding down the hall and out into the sunshine.

"Mom! Mom! Did you hear? He said I would be able to ride again!"

I stared at my feet keeping time with hers on the dusty sidewalk. I had to blink away the moistness in my eyes. I looked over at Nancy walking beside me. The sun touched her light brown hair and brightened the blue of her eyes.

"Yes. I heard." I pushed aside a wisp of hair on her forehead as I had done the first day she went off to school.

"I heard." To myself I added, *If all goes as planned. If...*

TWENTY FOUR

Graduation

For the first time in many months we talked. Really talked. Excitedly. Hopefully. The surgery would cause a year or more delay in Nancy's life, but after that there would be college as planned. Even horseback riding, *if all went as scheduled.*

How wonderfully good life was.

I hoped my optimism was well-founded. I also knew in life there were always elements of chance, of change, and especially of risk. Harrington Rod surgery was a major undertaking, lengthy and irreversible. Nancy's whole future depended on the skill of her orthopedic surgeon and on us.

I took Nancy for numerous rounds of x-rays and evaluations. So many factors had to be reviewed, including the strength of her lungs and heart. It was an exhausting several weeks, but Nancy good naturedly withstood all the poking and prodding, x-rays and tests.

One evening in May, Fred and I sat on our patio after supper, enjoying our coffee. For once, Nancy sat with us and we watched in awe as flock after flock of white egrets flew overhead toward their nightly resting spots. When the last bird had disappeared into the deepening sky, Nancy spoke.

"Mom, I was just thinking."

"Yes?" I rubbed my napkin over a coffee ring on the patio table, then started to gather up the mugs to take into the house.

"I was thinking," she hesitated, raised the chaise to a sitting position, then continued, "Let's go to Sanibel before my surgery. I won't mind July ninth so much if we just have a week on the island. Do you think we can?"

She turned to her father. "You wouldn't mind, would you, dad?"

He smiled, knowing when he was licked. But it gave

him a sense of fatherliness to be asked.

"You really wouldn't mind, would you?" she repeated.

He gave her a wink and shook his head. At that, Nancy jumped up for the chaise, wrapped her arms around his shoulders and squeezed hard. "Oh, daddy, daddy. Thank you, daddy."

The next day I called and made reservations for the week of June thirteenth, for a second floor studio apartment with a balcony overlooking the Gulf of Mexico.

There were still many things happening before then, though. Graduation parties, the Valhalla banquet and the Senior banquet, then graduation day.

What she wore to the banquets was an important subject. She sketched a dress similar to one she had found in *Seventeen* magazine, which, if purchased at one of the better stores, would have cost well over forty dollars. The material for the black crepe of the skirt and white for the bodice, plus the special daisy for the V-neck, cost us all of eight dollars.

On May nineteenth, Nancy came into the living room where Fred and I sat and she modeled her creation. I was proud of her and her workmanship.

"Mom? Dad? How do you like it?" She turned around before us.

"It's beautiful," I said.

Fred opened his eyes wide and grinned as he usually did when he approved.

The dress did look stunning on Nancy's slim figure and the black skirt hid the unevenness of her hips.

"Do you think anyone could tell I made it?"

"Not at all," I answered.

"Good."

With a swish she was off down the hall to her room to fix her hair. Twenty minutes later, two fellows from the Valhalla Yearbook staff came by to pick her up. I stood in the doorway, watching them hurry down the walk to the car.

Having made her decision to have surgery, she seemed to be returning to the happy young girl she used to be.

Her biggest disappointment of that year was not having a date for her senior prom. She confided in me that she had finally gotten up the courage to ask a boy in her art class, but someone else had already asked him. Prom night she baby-sat for a young couple across the street. I am sure she was trying not to think about what she was missing. I waited up for her to come home; wanting somehow to comfort her, but she quickly walked to her room and closed the door. I later heard her crying softly.

Graduation day, June eighth. The day we parents all dream of, when our children completed a part of their lives. More than any other event, high school graduation was a dividing line between childhood and adulthood.

I felt the excitement throughout our home. Nancy's white cap and gown hung on her closet door. Flowers arrived from friends and relatives in New England, joining the many cards and gifts from others close by. Nancy's childhood was just about over. Or, had it ended the day she made the decision to have surgery? I would never know. One thing I did know. Facing the next year or more would take maturity.

At two o'clock in the afternoon, Fred and I sat in the balcony of the large hall where eleven hundred students were to be graduated. Below us they began to march in and seat themselves, row after row. White gowns. White caps. White tassels. Young steps. Youth, so beautiful, so promising.

We focused our eyes on the fifth row. There, there she was, as she had said she would be. Minutes passed. Speeches and more speeches. Finally, the diplomas were handed out. Our eyes followed her every move. She stood up with the rest of her row and walked slowly toward the stage. When her name was called, Nancy stretched her five feet eight inches as tall and straight as she could and went forward to receive her diploma.

My eyes misted, my throat was tight and I touched Fred's arm, then folded my hands in my lap and prayed, "The Lord is the strength of my life. Let Him be hers also."

TWENTY FIVE

Preparing For Surgery

After our seven days on Sanibel, we returned home and began preparing for Nancy's surgery.

The next morning, after unpacking, Nancy came to me in the kitchen, holding the black shell box, with our precious two Angel Wing shells.

"Mom?"

"Yes?"

"Where should we put this? The bookcase in my room is filled."

"Hmm. What about the maple divider in the living room? That would be a good place. Then everyone can enjoy them."

"That's perfect! I want everyone to see them."

Yes, I thought, the Angel Wings should be shared.

Each morning I counted off the days. Nineteen. Eighteen. Seventeen days left until July ninth. Each night in bed, I chalked off another. I laid in the dark, wondering how the surgery would change our lives.

I was sure of Nancy's ability to endure. She was a plucky kid. But, could I stand the test? At forty-four, I figured my job as parent was almost over. Things were supposed to ease up as we approached the middle years, time to look forward to days of relaxation. One fact remained. I took my job as a parent seriously and never would stop being one. When Nancy was in need, I tried my best to fill it. My own mother still worried about my needs. How could I be any less a parent to my own child, regardless of her age, regardless of mine?

Nancy would need me. She would need her father and the assurance of family and friends. In the months to come she would need all of us.

There was one more thing Nancy was determined to do before her surgery. Her driver's exam. On the way to her appointment, she chattered nervously.

"I'm so glad I applied before July ninth. Afterwards it would be a long time before I could. And maybe they wouldn't even give it to me."

"Why on earth, not?" I asked.

She hesitated. "Maybe they'd think I was a bad risk because of my back."

Her words hit me hard. She was already having little doubts about *"after"* and the changes that would take place. The acceptance or rejection by others because she would have steel rods in her back. I hadn't given that angle much thought. She had triggered a doubt. Would she encounter problems after the fusion? Problems, not physical, but social? Right now, who would know about her back except someone who looked closely? Afterward, she would not be able to hide the fact of surgery. How much of a difference would it make?

I tried to reassure her, but she shrugged her shoulders. "Ehh, so what's the difference," she said in pretending nonchalance.

I waited as Nancy took her written test, then her road test. The inspector came to me afterward.

"A fine job," he said. "Your daughter handles a car well."

On the way home, Nancy chattered on, this time her nervousness gone.

"Gee, did you see how I did on my parallel parking? I backed into the space like nothing. Neat. Bet I couldn't do it again. Did you see?"

"Yes. You did fine."

"Pure luck. That's what it was. Pure luck."

"Oh, I don't know. I think it was more than luck."

In the days left, Nancy took full advantage of her license.

"Mom, you don't need your car today, do you?" Her familiar words were repeated often in the following weeks. She and Steph had plans for a beach party, or shopping, or a ride to the stables.

One day she came home smelling of horses. She showered, changed, and brought her grungy jeans out to the utility room where I was sorting laundry.

"I told Lester about the operation, mom. How I'm not supposed to ride much until way afterward. He wondered why he hadn't seen me much lately." She dropped her jeans on the washer.

I picked them up and started to put them into the metal tub. The inner sides of the legs were black with horse sweat. They were worn and faded, having straddled the flank of a horse more times than I could count.

How many sudsings had those old jeans gone through? How long before I again had to wash jeans that smelled like that? How long? I wondered.

The days passed all too quickly, but I knew we couldn't hold them back. I had always felt that work was an antidote for boredom or apprehension. So, I worked. Nancy helped. We cleaned house thoroughly, then sorted out closets and drawers, stacking clothes Nancy had outgrown, clothes she would never wear again. By the time we finished we had a half dozen bags of clothing stacked in the hallway, all clean, mended and still wearable.

Nancy and I packed the trunk full and drove forty miles down to the Perrine Migrant Mission. I had read several articles on the fine work the Mission was doing to help the migrants find a more stable life. I even thought of doing research and writing an article myself.

At the Mission we were greeted by volunteers who helped us unload all the bags of clothes and we placed them in the room next to the pastor's study.

The pastor greeted us, thanking us for our donation. He told us how, with encouragement from the Mission, some of the migrants were staying in the area. With steady jobs, they were able to keep their children in the church's day school.

He turned to Nancy. "How would you like to come and work with the children this summer?"

She leaned against the door casing. "I'd love to, but on July ninth I'm having an operation."

I could tell he didn't want to pry, but he was concerned. "I'm so sorry. Perhaps when you've recuperated?"

Nancy lowered her eyes and stared at her sandals as she made a circle on the scuffed floor. "It'll be a long time. A year. Maybe more. I'm having a spinal operation."

"I am so sorry." He glanced at me. I nodded. "I shall be thinking of you on July ninth. Next Sunday we shall say a prayer for you here, that God will guide you through your operation and long afterward."

Nancy bit her lip. "Thank you. I'd like that."

I swallowed hard and turned away. I could see the old sanctuary filled with tired old men and women, with weary sighs and creaking bones, praying for Nancy in Spanish or broken English. Praying for someone they didn't even know.

We were quiet all the way home that afternoon. We had been touched so deeply it hurt inside. What was there for us to say? The pastor had said it all. People did care.

Sunday, July 4, three days before Nancy was to check into the hospital, we went to a barbecue at Bette and Dick's.

Cousin Marilyn called out from the pool area, "Hi, Nan! Get on your bathing suit!"

"Hiya kid!" Steph's voice came up from the water and her blonde head appeared.

Soon Marilyn, Steph and Nancy made a threesome by the pool. Marilyn, at fourteen, was sprouting tall and lean like Nancy. Everyone could tell they were cousins. Stephanie was chunkier, solid, always grinning, her blonde hair braided into two sleek braids which fell below her shoulders.

"Come on! Race you to the other end!" she called. That was Steph. Always in action.

Poised at the deep end of the pool, the three girls dove in. I watched from the edge. Swiftly they moved their bodies underwater. Nancy and Steph took the lead, gliding gracefully forward. We never did decide who was the official winner. They broke the water together, flicked their heads and continued laughing, playfully pushing and ducking one another. No worries. No past. No future. Just the fun of right now.

Later we munched on hot-dogs and hamburgers smeared with mustard and ketchup. We ate our way through a platter of potato salad and polished off a pot of baked beans. Marilyn's reserved tone of voice, Nancy's soft responses, Stephanie's giggles remained in my mind long afterward.

July seventh, Nancy was scheduled to be admitted to Variety Children's Hospital. I wanted to transform the morning into an eternity. I scrambled eggs, made sure the toast was golden brown, buttering the slices slowly. Fred, Nancy and I sat at the dining table, forcing words. Nancy stirred her fork around in her plate, making hills and valleys with her food.

"Honey, eat," I said. Jabbing at my own plate, I placed a forkful of eggs into my mouth. I knew they were good, but they tasted like nothing. Fluffs of nothing. I swallowed and could feel them go all the way down. Nancy still sat, stirring.

"Please eat," I said again.

"Don't force her," Fred scolded in his usual soft way. "She's not a baby anymore."

"That's right, dad. You tell her."

"Hi!"

We heard a familiar voice and knock on the front door. In seconds, with a giggle and a grin, Steph moved into the room and plunked herself down in the chair beside Nancy. She reached over for a slice of bacon still on Nancy's plate.

"Why didn't you eat it, kid?" she said as she stuffed the slice into her mouth.

"Oh, no. Not you, too. Mom's been bugging me enough."

"Okay. Okay. So, don't eat it. I will." Stephanie took the last slice.

We laughed. The tension was finally broken.

"Come on. Picture taking time." Fred pushed his plate back and got up.

"No, dad. Not yet. Wait until I dress."

Nancy slipped out of her chair and hurried down the hall. When she returned, she had on the blue and white dress she had worn that day to Dr. Keiser's office. She had brushed her hair back casually.

Out on the back lawn, the two girls stood together in the warm summer sunshine. Steph's pigtails were fastened with two green elastics and her print blouse hung down over her shorts. The top of her head was level with Nancy's eyes.

"Hey, Mr. Webster. Get this!"

Stephanie grinned, her eyes pixie like. Nancy parted her lips and said the word cheese softly. Fred snapped the shutter.

That afternoon, Fred, Nancy and I rode south on the Palmetto Expressway toward the hospital. I don't know what Nancy and Fred's feelings were, but I'm quite sure they paralleled mine. Turmoil. I felt my insides spinning round as if I had a millions spheres inside me, in my stomach, my head, my heart. I felt tight in the middle of my chest, the only spot that wasn't spinning.

Straight. The word kept going through my mind. In two days Nancy would be straight.

At the hospital we went through the admitting procedure. The questions. The papers to be signed. The waiting. At last Nancy was assigned a room in the teenage section of Taylor Pavilion. She chose the bed by the window and before we knew it she was dressed in her hospital gown, sitting on the edge of the bed. Nurses buzzed around, going about their routines. I knew Fred and I were in the way.

"We'll see you during visiting hours tonight," I said.

"Okay, mom. Okay, dad." Nancy feigned lightness in her tone of voice and blew us a kiss.

On the way home my thoughts were racing. Fred's voice caught up to them.

"Honey, it's going to be rough."

"I know. I hate to see her have to go through this."

"I don't mean rough on her alone." Fred stared at the road ahead. "I mean it's going to be rough on you."

"You too," I replied.

"Not so much me. I'll do what I can, of course. But, you'll have to be with her constantly. You're her mother. She'll need you most of all."

I saw the tiredness in his face, a worry not there before. I touched his shoulder.

"I guess we'll just have to take it one day at a time, huh?" I rubbed my cheek on his arm. "It won't be so bad. Wait and see."

TWENTY SIX

New Beginnings

Answers? Would there ever be any? The more I searched, the more questions I had. Looking back over all the years, the only answer that made any sense to me was the possibility Nancy had contracted a mild case of polio. But no doctor would ever confirm it.

Christmas 1965 approached.

What a joyous holiday we looked forward to having that year! Nancy relished in decorating our Christmas tree, carefully unwrapping each treasured ornament, taking time to choose just the right spot to hang them on the tree. The full meaning of God's love lighted our home and our hearts as we watched her reach up, ignoring the slight hindrance of the chin rest on her cast, and place the star at the top of our tree.

I made a special Christmas dress that fit over Nancy's walking cast and she spent extra time fixing her hair and applying light makeup. Nancy carefully wrapped the sweater she had knitted for her dad. And, to my surprise, she had knitted a beautiful beige sweater for me. How she managed that, I am not quite sure.

We planned a big dinner with my mother and brother, who had traveled south for the winter. I spent several days beforehand baking extra pies and cookies. Christmas morning I put a big sixteen-pound turkey, with plenty of stuffing, in the oven. Along with it I prepared mashed potatoes, gravy, butternut squash, creamed onions and homemade rolls from Aunt Kate's recipe; all of our favorites.

Nancy helped set a beautiful table with my favorite china dishes and silver. As we sat down to eat, we all held hands and bowed our heads in prayer, thanking God for his bountiful love and guidance. Relatives, friends and neighbors began stopping by later in the day to share with us in giving thanks and to celebrate new beginnings.

January 1966. A new year and new beginnings!

We had reached the six-month point in Nancy's recovery and I called to schedule her appointment to have her walking cast removed. January 13 we returned to the Dr. Keiser's office in Coral Gables. The process this time was not quite as scary either to Nancy or to me, although the cast cutter saw sounded just as loud. Nancy lay on the examining table as the vibrating saw cut through her second cast.

When she stood up, draped in a white gown, the nurse said, "Watch her. She could be dizzy."

I was one step behind as she shuffled into the x-ray room saying, "I'm falling apart! Without my cast, I'm falling apart! Honest!" Her lightness of tone broke the tension of the climax of six months of waiting.

X-rays were taken of her back to ensure that she was progressing as she should. Her cooperation had paid off. There had been no slippage since the surgery. Dr. Keiser was pleased with her recovery and sent us directly over to an appointment with a specialist close by. He took Nancy's measurements for her brace she would be wearing for the next three to six months. For the next several days, until the brace was ready, Nancy had to be very careful how she moved and how long she sat.

We returned to the specialist and he strapped the brace around Nancy, showing us how each strap and snap should be placed and how much to tighten it. Although not nearly as confining as either the body cast or walking cast, it was quite an ordeal to get the straps and snaps in place, making sure it fit tight and secure around her back. Each morning, as soon as Nancy finished her shower, I helped her into the brace. She wore it until she was ready for bed each night. She never once complained, at least not out loud, of having to wear it, knowing it was the last step in her recovery.

With months left before Nancy could drive a car again or start college, filling time became a new challenge. During the week she divided her time between Steph's and

Pam's. Several days a week I drove Nancy over to Pam's to spend the afternoon and evening, the girls comparing their "rod" stories.

While Nancy was away from the house, I continued with my writing, finishing several chapters of my proposed book, *Two Angel Wings.* I joined several creative writing classes, eager for the completed chapters to be critiqued.

One Sunday, as Nancy was preparing to go to the beach with Steph, she remarked, "It's not icky enough." She fingered and pulled the once white sweatshirt down and out, completely out of shape.

I suggested if she wanted to wear a warm sweatshirt, she should take a better one. "This one has rust spots and look, a hole in the back. Don't you want to look neat?" I asked.

"Heavens no," she said. "I'd look out of place. This is just perfect. Besides, it covers my brace, so nobody can tell I'm wearing it."

By now she had the size thirty-eight pulled into a questionable forty-two or so, a size she couldn't possibly fill out even with her brace securely in place.

"I was out of place yesterday," she said. "Even Steph wore icky stuff."

She'd worn her fresh, starched gingham shorts and new top, just large enough to camouflage her brace. A beautiful combination and the way I thought an eighteen-year-old should look. The fit had shown off her wonderfully straight back. Now the old sweatshirt hung down, flopping off her shoulders.

"All the kids go there and they dress like this," she added.

There was a part of the beach where the surfers gathered, and the girls flocked to watch.

"And there's this man. They call him Holy Joe. He goes to all the beaches on Sunday, preaching to the kids. They just stand around and listen to him, and make fun of him sometimes."

"You're not going to make fun of him, are you?"

"No. I just want to go and see. I've heard the kids talk about him. He tells them they're all sinners and should repent and go back to the ways of the Lord."

"He's a self styled preacher?"

"Yeh, I guess."

"All right. Go. Wear the sloppy sweatshirt. Be with the other kids and watch the surfers. Listen to Holy Joe, but please, listen with your eyes and heart open. Don't be a part of the ridiculing. Besides, Holy Joe may have a very good point. Try to see his side of it. He's doing something that obviously he feels God appointed him to do, so remember sincerity and purpose deserve respect, even when you stand in a different corner."

Later that day Steph dropped Nancy off, sunburned, wrinkled and shaggy from beaching it. Her beach bag and towel trailed sand as she walked in.

"Whew. I'm tired."

"Did you see Holy Joe?"

"Yeh..."

"Well? Tell me."

"Oh, the kids were so mean. They're really a bunch of rough ones. Some of them dressed like this," she waved her arm down over herself, as if suddenly she couldn't stand how she looked.

"They threw sand at him and one kid put a lighted cigarette in his pocket. But he just stood there, preaching, *"Repent and be a child of God."* It was awful the way they laughed at him. I felt so bad for him."

"You didn't laugh, did you?"

"Oh, no. Steph and I just stood back and watched. He didn't seem to pay any attention to their shouting. And then he gave out these." She took a small pocket edition of the New Testament from her beach bag and handed it to me. "All over the beach. The kids threw them all over the beach and even tore some of them up."

"The Holy Bible? They tore up the Holy Bible?"

"Yes. They don't care. It doesn't mean anything to them."

I couldn't mask my horror that in 1966, in America, any youngster would lack respect to a point where he'd tear up the Holy Bible.

"It was sort of frightening," Nancy continued. "To see him keep on preaching and the kids trying to hit him. It was weird and I didn't like it."

"Now you saw it," I said. "You saw ridicule, which has no place in our lives. It's a cruel thing to see and no one is justified in practicing it. You didn't get overtired, did you? Your back. You're all right aren't you?"

"Oh, sure, mom. I'm okay. Just tired."

She headed for her room and a fresh supply of clothes for her shower.

I opened the small pocket Bible. The pages were new, but some stuck together. I flipped through, stopping for some reason on a page from the Second Epistle of Paul the Apostle to Timothy.

That the man of God may be perfect...

That our Nancy may be perfect. Perfection of mind and body, of heart and soul. Perfection seldom attained. Nancy was not perfect in body or mind. She, like all of us, was an erring human being, trying for perfection. I was sure though, that in picking up the little Bible, she had tried to cross out the disrespect shown that day on the beach.

It seemed her faith was being tested in many different ways.

In mid April we let Nancy travel with her church group to Stetson University in Deland to attend her Young Women's Convention. We felt she would be safe, not only because it was her church group, but Pam would be there too.

When she returned I was surprised to hear her slam the front door closed.

"Mom! Mom!"

"In the den," I answered, not sure of what was going on.

Her head poked around the door to the den, her face flushed with anger.

"I'm so glad you're my mother," she began. "I'm so glad you'll sit down and listen to me. And we're so mad, so mad. We wish we could start the whole day over and do it right this time. Not that we feel we did anything wrong, but we should have done it differently."

"Okay. Okay. Slow down and tell me all about it." I followed Nancy into her bedroom, where she dropped her suitcase on her bed.

Barely taking a breath, Nancy continued, "But for

her to almost insinuate that we were tramps. She said we'd lost our reputations and would be outcasts of the church. She wouldn't let us explain. And the boys, they just couldn't believe it. They kept saying, 'What did we do? We are so sorry, but what did we do?' And she told them, 'Just go along!' Imagine! She told them that we were going with her. She was so angry. We tried to explain to her that we were late for church because the boys had to go back to their dorm and change. But she wouldn't listen."

"Perhaps she thought you went into the dorm with them. You know with all the talk these days about college kids and frequenting the dorms and all that goes on. And don't forget you were her responsibility and she was worried."

"But Mom, we didn't even go into the dorm! We stayed outside and waited for them. And she didn't have to say she didn't even want to talk about it. So, later, after church, she said we could go for hot cocoa and the boys were there so we went over to talk to them and explain it all to them that she wouldn't let us go out with them. But then she walked in to check on us, saw us with the boys and made us go back to the motel. And then she came in and slept in our room! Stayed right with us to keep her eye on us! I was so furious I was shaking. I'm not a tramp and I don't understand what she thought we were going to do. Mom, you know I wouldn't lie to you. I just don't understand her being so unreasonable. She lets the rest of the girls have dates and you should have seen what they were doing around the pool. They were making out!"

"Making out? Good heavens. What does that mean?" I said, expecting the worst.

"It means kissing and hugging. Church. I'll never join that church, or any church. I'm disgusted."

"Disgusted? Why?"

"Because they say they're Christians and they won't even listen. She wouldn't even listen."

"Look honey. Churches are made up of individuals who are first of all human beings. Because they are church members doesn't mean they've cast of hypocrisy and have become perfection. They still have faults and failings. We all make mistakes. Growing up is learning to accept the fact that we are imperfect. Growing up also has a lot of disillusionment connected with it, but that will gradually give way to a deeper understanding and the ability to make allowances. You girls did make a mistake. You were with her and she was your chaperone. No matter what, you should have done what she said. Made every effort to be at the church when you said you would."

With a big sigh, Nancy opened her suitcase and started unpacking. I left her to think about what I had said.

Several days later, Nancy dressed for her church meeting.

"So, you are going?" I asked.

"Yes, mom," she smiled.

"I'm glad. You girls must understand that if we didn't care about you we wouldn't be so strict. You have so many things to face and get through. I remember back to things I did, actually, things I hope you will never do. And only by the Grace of God did they not backfire on me. This is a new beginning in your life. A trying period, so many awakenings, so many doubts, joys, miseries, hopes all intermingled. Just know that we love you. And your church group leader loves you. That's why she cared enough to see that nothing happened to you last weekend. It may have been all right, the boys many have been fine, nice boys, with only good intentions, but a half hour of talk is not enough to judge a boy and trust him enough to go with him. Now, be careful and enjoy your meeting."

"Love you, mom."

"Love you, too."

TWENTY SEVEN

Letting Go

In late April I took Nancy back to Dr. Keiser for her scheduled check up. After her exam and x-rays, we sat in his office waiting for her results. He came in holding her x-rays, another doctor with him. Smiling, he looked over his dark rimmed glasses at us.

"Her curves are holding at 10/25." He held up her x-rays for us to see. And what a fascinating sight. The long left distraction rod went almost the whole length of her incision. The right compression rod was shorter. He motioned Nancy to stand up.

"I want to show a disbeliever." He followed the line of her back, showing the other doctor the change from the original curvature to the straightness that she now had. His pride was obvious.

An idol? He certainly was an idol to all of his "children." Pam had come with us, waiting in the outer room, hoping to get a chance to see him again. To Nancy, there was no one more wonderful than Dr. Keiser, who had given her a straight back. Without him and the surgeries he had performed, Nancy and Pam's futures would have been uncertain.

"Now," he said. "You may go without your brace. You may swim, you may dance. No high diving or gymnastics though. Don't try and bend too far yet."

Yes! We were over the worst of it. Swimming? I could just see her back in the pool at Bette and Dick's, gliding through the water.

The next day, she and Pam were off to the beach with my car, fortified with a bag of oatmeal cookies and one dollar and ten cents between them. The dollar for tuck-away emergency money, the dime for parking.

"No bananas?" I asked.

"Heavens no," Nan replied. "We'd look like a couple

of monkeys sitting on Haulover Beach chomping on bananas."

To realize we must, and then to actually let go of our daughter was not as easy as we thought it would be. Throughout the whole time of enjoying this child that God as they say, had only lent us, we thought we were preparing. Not really. No one was ever fully prepared for separation.

Though Nancy was still our child and always would be, and she still lived under the protection of our home, she, indeed was beginning to leave us. Breaking away, that final pull from infancy and childhood into adolescence, then young maturity and young adulthood. Even the past months of surgery, casts and braces had only been a momentary slowdown in the natural process.

When before she had followed alongside, sharing in whatever we did, there was now a distinct cutting off. One afternoon at the public library, she tried so hard to control her impatience in what I was doing. Yet, I knew she wanted to be on with it and away. She was beginning to test her wings and they were carrying her off with her crowd.

"Mom, Pam and I just want to go to Scotties for some ice-cream." Or, "Mom, Steph and I are going to McDonald's for hamburgers. All the kids are going." Or, "Mom, I'm sorry I can't go with you. I promised I'd go with Pam and Linda to the Junior College for lunch."

Not long after Nancy came to me and asked, "Mom? Will you take me back to the stables? I want to see Lester and my friends, just to see how they are doing. Maybe Lester will let me sit on a horse for a few minutes?"

I knew the day would come when she would ask the question and I wondered how I should answer. If I took her back, she knew she couldn't ride yet, shouldn't even sit on a horse for even a few minutes. How hard would it be for her to watch the classes that she so dearly loved? If I didn't take her back, how much worse would that be for her?

Sixteen horses and their teenage riders circled the ring, walking, trotting, cantering, perfecting their figure-eights. Lester came over to us, hung his arm over the rail, smiling and with a little twinkle in his eyes.

"Well, hello, Nancy! We haven't seen you in a long

time. My, how you've grown!"

"Yeh. Over two inches in four hours. My spinal operation, you know."

"Yes, I remember. And how are you?"

"Fine." She gazed longingly at the riders passing in front of her.

The warmth of the sun touched down on us as we stood by the white fence, smelling the earth, the sweat of the horses, the leather of the saddles.

"It will be a while, quite a while before Nancy can ride again," I said.

"That's all right," Lester replied. "Nancy will pick up fast. She won't lose too much. We'll see to that."

Nancy gripped the white rail of the fence as if she were going to hoist herself up and over and into the ring. That was where her heart was. Riding, holding the reins firmly in her hands. Her riding boots stood in her closet, untouched. Her ribbons and mementos were tucked away in a storage box under her bed. But the memories couldn't be forgotten.

After class, Lester's son Ricky walked over and asked Nancy if she wanted to help groom one of the horses. Nancy's eyes lit up and she followed Ricky into the stables. He stood at the horse's head, holding the halter as she curried and brushed one of the horses. It certainly wasn't like being on a horse, but I know it must have helped a little.

In May Nancy asked if she could start driving again. Fred agreed that it was time, but wanted to drive with her a few times to observe her driving skills and how she reacted to situations. When he was satisfied that she felt comfortable behind the wheel, we let her go. The first time she drove off in my car by herself, I said my prayers. A prayer of thanks that she had finally reached this point and a prayer to keep her safe. Only an accident or severe jar could cause her rods to slip now. An accident, driving late at night, young people with their preoccupation's. A split second was all it took. All life hinged on that split second.

I worried each time she said, "Bye, mom!" I always ended my goodbye with, "And drive carefully!"

In June Nancy took her first class at Miami-Dade

Junior College. She wanted to get her feet wet after having been away from school and studying for over a year. On her first day she drove off in my car with the Miami-Dade sticker on the back window and her high school graduation tassel hung over the rear view mirror. She breezed through the class with a 4.0 and in the fall signed up for a full load, deciding to major in early education. She thrived on the challenge of new classes, keeping up an almost perfect grade point average, making new friends and beginning to date. She was emerging into the happy, vibrant young woman we knew she had the potential to be.

Of course, there were still trials along the way. One afternoon Pam joined Nancy and I on our back porch for lunch.

Pam began choking on her words, "An invalid. That's what she said we'd be, Nancy. Invalids all our lives because we had this spinal operation. She even said that Ken ought not to ever think of marrying me, because I'd always be complaining about my back."

"An invalid. For Pete sakes, I don't think I'm an invalid," Nancy answered. "I mean, sure, I can't bend, or ride horseback for a while, or take physical education when I start Junior College full time. But I'm no invalid."

Both girls looked at me.

I chose my words carefully. "No. You're not invalids as long as you tell yourselves you're not. And even if you were prevented for the rest of your life from indulging in all the activities you liked, you still wouldn't be invalids. Invalidism is a thing of the mind, not of the body. But you will be able to be active soon, in time that is, if all goes as planned. And so far it has for both of you. What this well meaning woman was unconsciously trying to plant in your minds was an indulgence far worse than any other, that of self-pity. Never, never indulge in that, for it is one of the most crippling of emotions. But, I really don't need to tell either of you any of this. You are both young, full of life, and above all filled with faith."

TWENTY EIGHT

Thunderbolt

"There's a lady coming to call on us Wednesday evening," Fred said in his casual way.

"A lady? Why?" I asked. I looked over the dining table beyond the flickering candles.

"Just a lady," he said, spearing his fork into the apple pie I had baked just hours before. His thinning light brown hair seemed to be an extension upward of the candle glow. His blue eyes laughed in the mysterious, quiet way I knew indicated something was going on.

"Come, on. Tell me. What lady and why is she coming to see us?"

"Oh," he continued in his slow steady voice. "I dropped by Stone Realty this afternoon and told them we wanted to sell the house."

"You what?" I swallowed, unchewed, a big chunk of apple.

"That is what you wanted, isn't it?" Now he grinned.

Nancy blurted out, "Dad, you did? Really, dad? How neat!"

"It is what you wanted, isn't it?" Fred repeated, looking from Nancy to me.

"Yes! Yes!" we both answered.

I had wanted this so much, I had almost given up hope that it would ever happen.

"Yes, we're going to sell and move to Davie," I began telling family and friends in the days following.

"How did you ever change his mind?" was the same question asked.

"I didn't," I answered. "He changed it himself."

And I remembered the turning point. April 23, Fred's birthday. We planned a big barbecue with family and friends on our lot in Davie. We sat in the shade of the melaleukas, grilled hot dogs and hamburgers, drank our cokes and beer. We looked through the grove of melakeukas to the spot where we dreamed our house would be someday. After the sun slipped down over the Everglades sawgrass, we watched the moon rise up over the fields and canal. We listened to frogs croaking and for the first time in over ten years we saw fireflies. The peace and quiet of that night reminded us that in this rushed, confused, hectic world, there still were places we could find tranquillity.

It seemed like we'd been through this once before. When we put our house on the market, the fun began. From the moment we signed agreements to sell and the agent picked them up in her hands, we had an inkling of what it would bring. People, we hoped, but not too many too early or late.

"You'll never do it," the man behind the counter in the building permit department said. He pushed his glasses back up his nose ridge with his forefinger. "Not for $8,500. It'll take at least $10,000."

"It better not," I answered. Standing firmly on my right foot, I rested my left heel down on it as I usually do when I am pondering a situation, or embarking on a big project.

For Fred, Nancy and me this was a big project.

"We're doing all the work ourselves," I continued, trying to convince him.

He shook his head. "Still won't do it." He wrote down a compromising figure of $9,000.

I paid the $55.00 fee and held the stiff white card-board permit that would allow us to begin our dream home in Davie. A modest two bedroom, one bath, New England style home, similar to the "old house." We knew what we wanted and how little we had for it. Much less than the $8,500 I had told the building board. Beyond our meager assets, we would work on faith and muscle and with time. $9.00 went for blueprinting the Fred's sketches. Then, another $25.00 went to a registered architect for carefully examining and placing his seal upon the prints.

We had spent many nights sitting at our kitchen table making sketches. *The living room goes here. The kitchen must have a Dutch door out to the breezeway. We'll find a cupola and weather vane for the top of the garage.*

The outside will be all wood shingles painted barn red with white window shutters. There will be a path leading from the lanterned drive up to the colonial front door with a big brass knocker.

We broke ground on May 27, 1967. We started clearing, raking, digging and building. Our North Miami home sold more quickly than we anticipated and we moved into mama's small 26x27 foot one room home which had been completed the previous year. Most of our furniture was in storage and we were undeniably cramped, but the prospect of our new home under construction gave us the patience to make it work.

Always the perfectionist, Fred supervised every aspect of the job and did most of the inside carpentry work himself. Fed wouldn't let me nail nails. I hadn't yet learned to nail them straight. However, I ordered materials, checked them on delivery, counting 2x4s and cement blocks, swept and cleaned up the sawdust and discarded nails afterward. We sported calluses and blisters. I learned quickly that concrete could skin my hands if I didn't use gloves. Cement blocks were heavy. Studs, roof trusses, sheathing, shingles, windows and doors all cost money. But putting them all together and creating our dream home was one of the greatest personal achievements of our life together.

We managed to recreate our "old New England Saltbox" complete with red shingles and white shutters, moving in late that fall. The only thing missing was a fireplace, but we later made up for that by adding a swimming pool. In our living room we found the perfect spot for Nancy's black shell box and our precious two Angel Wings.

I knew in my heart Nancy was still not ready to give up on her dream of having her own horse. After all, we lived in the middle of horse country. Most of the fields surrounding us were filled with horses of all colors and sizes. Knowing it was only a matter of time before the subject came up again, I was not surprised when one Saturday afternoon she approached her dad.

"Dad, can I show you something?"

Fred looked up from his paper, not sure of what she wanted.

"Dad, there's a horse and he's for sale. He's across the street in the pasture and the owner's there right now. Please, dad. Please, come see him?"

The three of us walked across our tiny bridge, across the road and into the pasture.

"Ride him," the owner said, saddling the strong, filled out body. "Try him out. He's a beauty. Has a smooth gate."

With hope in her face, Nancy hoisted herself into the saddle and placed her feet in the stirrups. Holding the reins firmly, yet with just enough slack, she nudged him with her heels. Off down the path they went, the horse balking a bit with a new rider on his back. He wanted to turn, but she let him know she was in the saddle. He bobbed his head in defiance, but did her bidding.

"What do you want for him," Fred asked.

"$175," replied the owner.

"Is he okay? I mean, shouldn't we have a vet check him?" I asked.

"If you want. He's okay, though. I know. And these people here want him too." He motioned to a family standing back watching.

"We'd better take him if we want him," Fred said. "Or, we'll lose him.

It was inevitable. Fifteen minutes later, we were owners of over a thousand pounds of horse. He was a beauty, a sorrel with a golden mane and tail and white patch from his forehead to his wet, snorting nose. He did have a smooth gait and a proud stance, his knees rose high in a fast trot or canter.

"Are you out of your minds?" one neighbor asked. He was one who didn't mince words. "Nancy's back! What if she should fall?"

We knew there was a danger. Maybe he was right. But there was danger in Nancy driving a car, too. Perhaps more so. How far could we go in being careful? To the point of withdrawing her from life?

Soon Fred fenced mom's back pasture in, adding a large gate with THUNDERBOLT painted in black letters on the white gate rail. Each morning, before her college classes, Nancy fed him. He knew the sound of the shed door opening and closing, knew his grain was coming. He would snort and pace back and forth along the fence as Nancy approached.

"Talk to me Thunder!" was Nancy's morning greeting.

He snorted louder and paced faster until she slid the bucket under the fence. She would stand and watch him munch away happily.

Each day after classes, Nancy drove home, took his bridle and bit and headed for the pasture. Some days, when she didn't feel like putting his saddle on, she rode bare back.

"Just be careful," I always said, knowing without the saddle she had less control and yet, in a way, had to prove she was a better rider.

"He's a spoiled devil," she said one afternoon after her ride. Thunder's body was wet. His ears turned back, then straight up, his nose circling the air.

"Spirited?"

"Spirited is not all of it. Spoiled. Spoiled and spirited." she answered. "Know what he did?"

"No, what?"

"Well, he won't let another horse get ahead of him, that's what. I was walking him down Cherry Road when he spotted some other horses way ahead. He just took off! There was no holding him. He galloped until he had passed them all. He's a devil! But a beautiful one." She leaned over to pat his lean neck.

He was unpredictable and stubborn. More than once Nancy had to use the ends of the reins on the top of his head to stop his antics, or apply a switch to his rump to move him along when he wanted to stop and graze.

One afternoon, Nancy decided to use just his halter. She jumped on his back and rode off. She told me later that Thunder was feeling especially rambunctious that day, bobbing his head, his strong, slim legs ready to break out into a gallop, his ears back then forward, balking at her restraint and mastery over him. He seemed to be conjuring up something different to try on her, to test her ability to win out. Trotting up the back lanes, he came to an abrupt stop when he reached a patch of soft sand. Without warning he went down on all four knees. Instinct and the quickness of youth made her slide off quickly and move out of the way. Thunder, completely unmindful of whether his mistress was on or off, began to roll, over and over, in complete delight, back and forth in the soft sand. There was no stopping him. Finally, when he finished with his sand scratch bath, he righted himself and stood up proud and victorious. He looked over at Nancy with a snort and a bob of his head.

Nancy laughed and said, "Okay, Thunder. You won this one." She grabbed the halter rope, swung up on his back and rode home again. When they rode into the yard, the smile on her face reminded me so much of the grinning four-year-old who, so many years before, had asked,

"A horse Daddy. Can I have a horse?"

EPILOGUE

It has taken me many years to accept the fact that, sometimes, there are no definitive answers to our questions. I simply must go on faith that there is a reason for everything.

For Nancy and me, our two Angel Wing shells remain our source of strength, our vessels of Faith, and we believe a force for good. Before any tough or challenging event or uncertainty we have facing us, we always say, "Remember the two Angel Wings."

In the summer of 1968, Dr. Keiser advised Nancy to have her Harrington Rods removed. Nancy asked and was given the rods as a reminder of her ordeal. On her last visit with her doctor, his parting words to her were, "I would advise not to try and have children. And most importantly, Nancy, don't do anything what would contribute to your falling."

Within four weeks of her surgery, Nancy was back riding Thunderbolt.

We did not return for our mother-daughter week on Sanibel Island until the summer of 1972. When we did, there were three of us walking along the beach searching for shells, myself, Nancy and Nicole, my precious two-year-old granddaughter.

We lost Stephanie on December 29, 1972. She was one of two flight attendants, along with so many, many others, whose lives tragically ended in the crash of Eastern Airlines flight 401 in the Everglades. Several days later, Stephanie's body was found face down, still strapped in her jump seat. I don't think Nancy has ever really accepted the loss of her "sister." Nancy's only way of coping is the firm belief that Stephanie is her Guardian Angel.

Stephanie was someone few people really knew. The outward Stephanie was bubbly, giggly, always smiling and laughing. Those who met her briefly might have considered her just another lovely young woman with a frivolous daring for life. Oh, she was that, lovely and daring, but not frivolous. There was a side to Stephanie only those closest to her were privileged to see.

Stephanie, the little eight year old with blond pig-tails, who came rushing into our yard the day we moved into our new home in Miami. On the patio that day in May, a friendship began which only became stronger as the years passed. Oh, it had its spurts of differences, its moments of apartness, but always they came back together and grew up together. Nancy and Stephanie. They could not have been more like sisters if they had had the same blood.

I will never forget the passage that Stephanie wrote in Nancy's high school yearbook:

Nan,

No matter what happens, we will always be best of friends and with luck and love from the Lord above, our children will grow up together and learn to find their eternal friend as I have found in you. Nancy, you know I will always be here when you need me. So just yell! God Bless you and our friendship for the rest of our lives.

Love always,
Steph

Made in the USA
Monee, IL
08 November 2026

67380516R00103